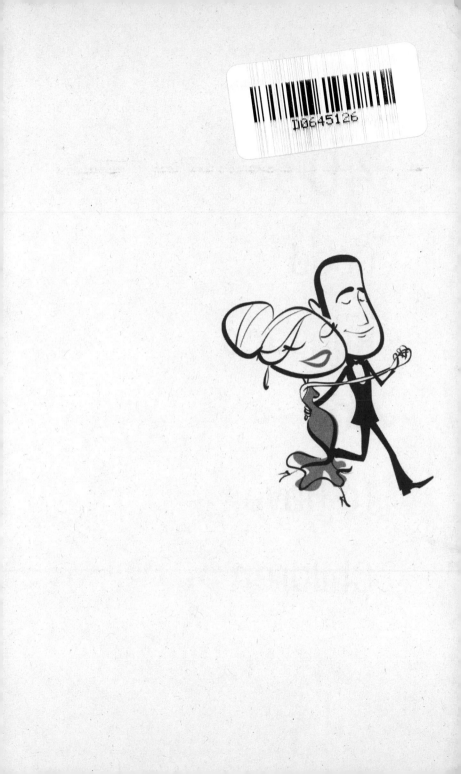

40

Good

Reasons

NOT

to Have

Children

Corinne Maier

Translated from the French by PATRICK WATSON

NO KIDS

3 1705 00387 0075

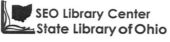
SEO Library Center
State Library of Ohio

40780 Marietta Road, Caldwell, OH 43724

EMBLEM

Original title: No Kid: Quarante raisons de ne pas avoir d'enfant
Copyright © 2007 by Éditions Michalon
English translation copyright © 2008 by Patrick Watson Enterprises Ltd.

Published under arrangement with Éditions Michalon, Paris, France
First English-language edition published in 2009 in Canada by McClelland & Stewart

All rights reserved. The use of any part of this publication reproduced, transmitted
in any form or by any means, electronic, mechanical, photocopying, recording, or
otherwise, or stored in a retrieval system, without the prior written consent of the
publisher – or, in case of photocopying or other reprographic copying, a licence from
the Canadian Copyright Licensing Agency – is an infringement of the copyright law.

Library and Archives Canada Cataloguing in Publication

Maier, Corinne
    No kids: 40 good reasons not to have children / Corrine Maier
    Previously published under title: No kid.
ISBN 978-0-7710-5477-8
    1. Childlessness I. Title
HQ 755.8.M337 2008   306.87   C2008-907110-7

We acknowledge the financial support of the Government of Canada through the
Book Publishing Industry Development Program and that of the Government of
Ontario through the Ontario Media Development Corporation's Ontario Book
Initiative. We further acknowledge the support of the Canada Council for the Arts
and the Ontario Arts Council for our publishing program.

Typeset in Electra by M&S, Toronto
Printed and bound in Canada

ANCIENT FOREST
FRIENDLY
This book is printed on processed chlorine-free paper that is 100% ancient-forest
friendly (40% post-consumer recycled).

McClelland & Stewart Ltd.
75 Sherbourne Street
Toronto, Ontario
M5A 2P9
www.mcclelland.com

1   2   3   4   5   13   12   11   10   09

CONTENTS

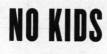

NO KIDS

Prologue

THE ONLY SOLUTION: CONTRACEPTION

In 2006, France became the fertility champion of Europe. The "French Miracle" was crowed about in victorious tones – *Cocorico!* Today in France we are seeing a glorification of maternity that would have made Marshal Pétain proud. It's the new face of patriotism: if we must deal with the hell of living, then the more the merrier.

Everyone, take warning from France's example. In this deathly boring and moralistic world, they want you to think that happiness is to be found in your two breasts, in making babies, and in your job. The truth is that the more your fecundity increases, the fewer there are of you who can call yourselves happy. Open your eyes! Your kids are going to be the "loser babies," destined for unemployment, or precarious or inferior jobs; in other words, factory drones. Their lives will be way less fun than yours, and that's saying a lot. Listen: your marvellous babies have no future because every child born in a developed country is an ecological disaster for the whole planet.

And you – you're going to spend twenty years of your life "raising" them. The education of children has become a sacrament: society demands of modern parents a level of performance worthy of Superman or Superwoman. Always on call, smiling, attentive, teacherly, and responsible – is there anything you won't do to guarantee the "happiness" and "fulfillment" of the kids? Becoming a parent means giving up everything else: your life as a couple, your leisure time, your sex life, your friends, and, if you're a woman, your career success.

All that for *kids*? Honestly, is it really worth it?

Take the necessary precautions. Having children – it happens too quickly. The only solution is contraception.

Introduction

One day in December, I was at café with a friend. My fortieth birthday was looming, and I was feeling down about it, and taking stock – having already taken a few drinks.

"I'm off track," I said to my friend. "I started my analysis ten years too late. I'm sick of dinners out with all these high-society types. I've never known how to grab destiny by the forelock (yes, I realize that destiny now has a Mohawk). My kids are driving me nuts. . . ."

"Listen," she said. "It's one thing to doubt your whole life at this point, but you're not *serious* about regretting having kids!"

"I'm totally serious. If it weren't for them, I'd be travelling around the world with all the money I've made from my books. Instead, I'm stuck at home, serving meals, getting up at seven o'clock in the morning every day of the week to help them with their homework and run the washing machine. All that for these kids who treat me like I'm their slave. Yes, some days, I'm sorry to say, I really regret it, and I'm not afraid to say it. When they were born, I was young and in love – and, of course, ruled by hormones. If I had to do it all over again, to tell you the truth, I'm not sure that I would."

She was shocked. There are some things that a *mère de famille* – the mother of a family – just doesn't say, or she risks being seen as a monster. The party line is, "I'm proud of my children: if there is *one* thing I do not regret, it's becoming a parent."

The Cult of the Child

Having a baby is the most beautiful thing in the world, a dream within reach of every wallet and every uterus. It is the outward and visible sign of a couple's success, the proof that the new parents have become part of society in a world where the greatest fear of all is to be "excluded." Children are the ultimate fashion accessory, and stylish people must always have a nursing child on the hip or a kid nestled in a stroller. As for pregnant women, nowadays they pose nude in magazines – pregnancy is no longer something you have to conceal. Maternity and parenthood have never been so celebrated.

The Great Adventure of the 21st century is unquestionably having children. The proof? John de Mol, the millionaire founder of *Star Academy* (and reality

TV itself), recently conceived the notion of filming a pregnancy from conception right through to delivery. They would show everything: the nausea, the ultra-sound, the medical tests, the weight gain, all the states of mind. . . . It would be unbearable and poignant suspense. Better than *The Bachelor*, *Survivor*, and *America's Next Top Model* rolled into one.

Here's a little flashback. At the dawn of civilization, mankind loved plentiful harvests, big breasts, fat buffaloes, and lots of kids. You had to populate the world, hunt, and dominate your quarrelsome neighbours – which is where the reverential respect fertility inspires today came from. When modern medicine reduced the risk of dying during childbirth, a new idea emerged in Europe, the *desire* to have children. Ever since the pill and the IUD, most of the children who have been born have been *wanted* children. They are no longer the unavoidable consequence of a sexual act but the product of willpower under scientific management. The unforeseen has been eliminated. Long live planning! Have the first child at thirty, when you finally have a steady job; the second when you buy a home; the third when you need to reduce your income taxes.

The desire for children gives carte blanche to short-sighted adults (and there are lots of them) to consecrate themselves body and soul to the blossoming of these amazing little creatures. For a lot of silly or naive people, the child, now totally sacramentalized, represents the missing link between the human and the infinite. It is not *Demain les chiens* (the French title of Clifford Simak's science fiction collection *City*), but *Today the Children*. Thomas Malthus, who preached population control toward the end of the 18th century, is seldom spoken of these days. Malthusians, their numbers dwindling, are seen as cynical anti-patriots, even as dangerous anarchists.

Pay attention: The more you are pro-birth, the sooner you die!

In 2006, the French press triumphantly announced that France was the most fecund country in Europe, with a record 830,000 births.*

Why were journalists so fascinated? Was it because more births would mean more activity on the stock exchange? Why was this a victory? Was it because that's all France has left to boast about? With this new "natalism" and "familialism" being so glorified, is

---

* In 2006, with a childbirth rate slightly above 2 children per woman, France indeed became, along with Ireland, the most fertile country in Europe. Belgium had a birthrate of 1.6 children per woman, and France's Italian, German, and Spanish neighbours had rates no higher than 1.4. Eastern European countries are facing a huge low-birthrate crisis, while childbirth rates in the U.S. are higher than in Europe, at 2.1 children per woman. Why? It is their way of showing "optimism" and patriotism, and their religious faith is stronger.

Philippe de Villiers actually in power right now?*

In our country, the norm is to want children. But it was not always so. For a long time, the French balked at the idea. From the 18th century up to the 1970s, they were demonstrably hostile to the idea of parenthood. The French birthrate was so low that some people were really worried about the survival of the national identity (though it was not yet called that). Today the French seem to have been infected by a strange fever. Everybody talks about the desire for a child as if it's a vital impulse surging up from deep within – irresistible, feverish, inexplicable, and completely justified. A lot of parents feel they are carrying out some kind of national mission, a sacrament that makes possible the holy and the transcendent. The child has become so exalted that making its own way in life is considered beneath it.

Everybody dreams of having a child. Gay couples want to adopt. Lesbian couples want to legitimately bring forth the fruit of their flesh, even if France's Civil Code doesn't recognize this as legitimate yet, since the law – enamoured of the "natural" – still considers real parenthood to be based on the body. But the right to have a baby is pushing its head up over the horizon, like the controversial right to housing, or the right to

---

* Head of the party Mouvement pour la France, the traditionalist, anti-Islam, Catholic Philippe de Villiers ran for president in 2006 and received just over 2 per cent of the vote. (Ed.)

happiness, the right to health, the right to be thin. What's next, an official declaration of the right to eternal childhood, allowing us to live forever in a fantasy world of wonder?

In France, as soon as you get married, your co-workers immediately start hounding you, asking, "So? Are you trying?" Some women even invent a child just so people will leave them in peace at the office, where this *diktat* of maternity, underpinned by a vigorous national policy (family allowances, daycares, preschools, and so on), is most strongly enforced. Among French women who have lived past menopause, only 1 in 10 has not had a baby. In Italy and Spain it is 14 per cent, in the U.K. 20 per cent, and in Germany 30 per cent – 45 per cent for those women who have a postsecondary education. But more and more, France is held up as an example to the rest of Europe: Germany has just instigated paid parental leave for a whole year. Europeans, get to your bedrooms! There is just one head we all want to see: your baby's.

The Mandatory Use of the Pacifier

The problem is that in the long history of the oppression of peoples (which is often confused, understandably, with History itself), a family with children has been a categorical imperative often on a par with work. There was that sinister slogan of Marshal Pétain's, "Work,

Family, Fatherland" (*Travail, Famille, Patrie*). "Get to work, reproduce yourselves, and then you will never think of doing anything you shouldn't do, and I shall take care of law and order." That is the unwritten rule of every dictator. The State has an interest in your having children: is that not a bit suspect? Is that not a good reason to question this "civic duty" to contribute to the renewal of the generations? It is, obviously, a matter of demographic obsession, intended to maintain some supposed world vision.

But the hackneyed old argument "Europe is aging; the renewal of the generations is in danger" doesn't stand up to scrutiny for one second. On the one hand, let's bring in immigrants to take the jobs our young people don't want (bricklayer, waiter, nurse), and on the other hand, let's finance people's retirement. There is no shortage of applicants for immigration: all we have to do is open the doors. As for the nonsense about the children of today being the growth of tomorrow . . . Growth? What for? Is economic growth the only legitimate purpose of a would-be democratic society? Are there no dreams beyond buying TVs, washers and dryers, and cellphones, just to provide mindless jobs that are an insult to everyone's intelligence, employers and employees alike? The tired line from the economists (often gentlemen of a certain age, long-winded and pretentious) is a joke. Economics (which claims to pronounce authoritatively on a reality that is in fact profoundly difficult to determine) has never impressed me. Listen, I've been calling myself an "economist" for years: I know all the tricks of this non-trade.

Fortunately, there are some conscientious objectors to this fertility mythology. I'm referring to the people who simply don't want kids. They are discreet, of course – they have to be. It's acceptable for women to delay having a baby, but to *refuse* to? No way. Lately, men are being told that they too will have wasted their lives if they don't father children. Tolerance for a wide variety of lifestyles may be growing, but to declare flatly that you don't want children, well, that's just inviting persecution. So universal is the value accorded to family that those who have the nerve to refuse parenthood are seen as social deviants. To be "childless" is considered a defect; irrevocably judged, those who have decided they just don't want children are also the objects of pity: "The poor thing; I guess she just wasn't able to," or "He has wasted his life." These "egoists," "adolescents," "pessimists," or "eccentrics" are crushed by the taxes imposed by a totally unjust fiscal system that gives preference to families, and are confined to the margins of a world where everything is dedicated to the dominant model. So what if some people have different ambitions? Everybody will tell them that those ambitions pale in comparison to the "joys" of having children, to the "self-fulfillment" that parenthood promises.

There is a commendable counter-offensive developing. In the 1980s, in the United States and Canada, Australia and England, "non-parent" associations began to appear. Having grown into genuine pressure groups, these associations now insist that the word *childfree* replace the derogatory *childless*. They see not having children as a choice, not a handicap. Their members don't feel deprived; they are quite happy, thanks very much.

Furthermore, some of these groups are saying out loud what many people believe quietly: that children are a pain in the ass. Hugh Grant has said of them, "I can't bear mess or ugliness and those things come hand-in-hand with children." He's the exception, though; can you imagine Angelina Jolie or Tom Cruise saying anything like this? In Florida there are childfree zones, subdivisions where under-thirteens are not allowed, communities for thirty-somethings who find the inconvenience of children intolerable. Across the United States and more recently in Scotland, retirement villages completely closed to children are cropping up – and are much in demand. The concept, it seems, is popular. So far these communities stay under the radar. The "childfree" promoters are too afraid of having stones thrown at them.

Discouraging potential parents

This little book is intended to further discourage those potential parents everywhere who are beginning to wonder if having children is really worth the trouble. Of course, they can't share their doubts with anyone: raising the question is simply not done, because *having children is good.* However, there is a multitude of excellent reasons not to have children, at least forty of them – reasons that are far more rational than the ones we usually come up with for having kids.

So enough of this vapid talk about the glory of parenthood. In the face of all the enthusiasm and obligatory fine sentiment, saying "bullshit" to nurseryland is urgent and necessary. And I speak from experience. I have kids. There are some things that only a *mère de famille* can say, if she has the nerve to come out and say them. If I had written this book *without* having had children, everybody would have accused me of being an embittered and jealous old hag. I expect I'll still be called an unworthy mother. First I publish my "treasonous" book *Bonjour Laziness,* now I am denouncing the picture-postcard image of the family that in truth exists only in magazines. I use it to make fun of the baby-obsessed, self-satisfied part of society, whose entire vision consists of work and reproduction. This is the real sign of a distressing regression: what could be more depressing than a society hell-bent on reproducing what it is now, when what it is now is already so depressing and deadly boring?

40

Good Reasons
NOT
to Have Children

1.
The "desire for children": A silly idea

Wanting to reproduce yourself at any cost is to aspire to the pinnacle of banality. I'll admit that there is a certain amount of security in behaving like everyone else and acting just like your neighbour. To be "accepted" in today's society means having a job, a baby, or both. Sign up, and then sign up again. The decision *not* to have a child is taken as an indication of such procreative bitterness that it defies comprehension. Reproductively obsessed people are expected to undergo fertility treatment with the determination of Olympic athletes. And with, it must be said, the complicity of doctors who find themselves a bit uneasy – who wouldn't be, working with a science that is always one step behind?

The craze for having children is so widespread these days that it has become a big business and is growing fast. Every day, ova, sperm, and babies are for sale, all over the world. Wombs are for rent, with a nine month lease. Specialty clinics are popping up planetwide; the price varies according to the "value" of the product: white babies cost more than black ones. In the United States, ova from a Columbia University student are worth more than those from a Harvard student. This "baby business" is less advanced in Europe, and doesn't yet exist in France at all, at least officially: the State here, set up to safeguard our "welfare" and our morality, is on the lookout.

"A child for everyone and everyone for a child" has given rise to all kinds of debate, all of it both tiresome and ridiculous. Choose sides, comrade: it's hard to tell which is worse, but easy to see that both are stupid.

On my left there's the so-called *right to a child*. This has become such a sacred trust, you almost expect it to turn up in the preamble to the Constitution. "The child" has become so indispensable, so miraculous, that everyone must exercise their right to it. But what about the right *not* to have a child, on the other side? To whom we would grant this right is unknown, but I suspect that the most industrious are going to find someone. I mean, take me: I no longer have parents; they're dead. Am I going to demand the "right to have parents"? Stage a hunger strike until some court or other decides to give me a new set (being unable to give me back the old ones, since science has not yet figured out how to bring the dead back to life)? No, let's be sensible: a child is neither a right nor a necessity – it's simply . . . a possibility.

The view to my right isn't much better. Having children seems to be the focus of a particularly depressing discussion in France: "A family in which a child's happiness is assured consists of a father and mother, period." That *two persons of the same sex* could adopt and raise a child, well, you wouldn't think the idea had ever entered our dear little blonde heads.* Opponents of gay parenthood would have everyone "abnormal" fall back into line. And that line will be formed by shrinks who will advise about anything and everything in the name of Oedipus, and by anthropologists who know everything there is to know about mankind. Politicians, of course, are already the first to use the child in order to control the population (no medically assisted pregnancy for single women, no access to fertilization treatments for gay couples, even though both are available in many other European countries). In short, as the singer Patrick Bruel put it, "*Who has the right?*" What *is* the "right to have a child," and who gave anyone the right to tell us what to do?

---

* The expression *nos chères têtes blondes* is a currently popular phrase in France and the title of a 2006 comedy directed by Charlotte Silvera. (Ed.)

2.
Labour is torture

The joys of giving birth? That's brainwashing. Except for the very few women whose bodies are tube-shaped, childbirth hurts. A lot. Yes, an epidural is an enormous help, but even with that the delivery itself is far from fun. Speaking for myself, it was the most painful thing I have endured in an admittedly sheltered life. Women who say, "Giving birth was the most beautiful moment of my life," always seemed suspect to me, and once I had actually gone through it, I knew they were lying. Some women will say, cautiously, "I don't remember a thing," which is just another way of saying, "I don't want to talk about it."

The reality is that a delivery takes hours, sometimes a whole day. You're immobilized like some giant beetle with a pin stuck through your back. The contractions make you feel like you're exploding. . . . Labour is pain, blood, and exhaustion (and shit, too, it seems, but that's a gift to the midwife or the doctor). You've seen the film *Alien*, where a monster rips its way out of the body of one of the characters through his stomach? Do you know why this scene is so memorable? Because it is very, very close to a real-life delivery.

But the worst part comes after the actual birth – the feeling of total exhaustion. The stretch marks on that poor stomach, which will never again be that of a young girl. The encounter with a messy little human creature for whom you are going to be responsible for an endless number of years. Michel Houllebecq, in *The Possibility of an Island*, writes of the "legitimate disgust that overwhelms a normally made man upon the appearance of a baby." In fact, a newborn infant is frighteningly ugly: red-faced and flushed, with no facial features, its eyes veiled with a bluish opacity – everything about it should fill us with revulsion. Yet more and more young parents are turning childbirth into a photo op, and don't seem in the least aware that they're the only ones (well, along with their own parents) who take any pleasure from those photos.

Society in general worships babies. Apparently it's the thing to do, to adore any human larva a few days old. I'm sick and tired of it, and when I admitted to my new-mom cousin that I don't have the least interest in newborns, she looked horrified, faced with this crime of *lèse-bébé*.* Enough with the babies! On TV, on billboards, they're everywhere – not, by the way, actual newborns, but rather the more presentable version that is already a few days old. And while we're glorifying babies more and more, old age and death are being hidden deeper away and feared. Is there a cause-and-effect connection here? Infantomania and gerontophobia –

---

* A play on *lèse majesté*, which means "high treason." (Ed.)

do they go hand in hand? Probably. Long live youth! Down with age, and especially death, which no longer means anything to us. Back in the 19th century, effigy-lovers were having a field day, painting and sculpting and photographing the dead. But today it is only the celebrity dead who appeal to us.

3.
You avoid becoming a walking pacifier

Professional baby-lovers all hammer the same thing into us: nursing your baby is fabulous. "Breast is best," as they say. Primal, natural, out in the open air, no pesticides, no genetically modified foods. Breastfeeding may have gone out of style in the '60s and '70s, but it's been back for a while, with a vengeance. Countless articles extol the benefits of breastfeeding. The baby will be "healthier" and have "fewer allergies," and of course "there's just no substitute for this bonding time with the child." In France, 60 per cent of new mothers are breastfeeding – for only a few weeks, of course. The public policy objective is to get that up to 70 per cent by 2010.

In case simple persuasion isn't enough to convince the rare holdouts – the "ill informed" – they're now being bribed with money. In 2003, the First Health Insurance Bank of Morbihan, in Brittany, decided to offer a "breastfeeding premium" to women who agreed

to nurse their babies for at least a week. What's next —
income-tax relief for nursing women? Why not a bonus
for every woman who refuses the epidural, since a delivery without anaesthetic is "more natural" and thus
probably "better" for the infant? When I told the maternity ward staff that there was absolutely no question
of my nursing my baby, the attendant looked at me
disapprovingly and told me that this was Not Good. A
month later, the gynecologist accused me of "refusing
to connect" with the baby. The noose is tightening on
those unworthy women who bottle-feed. Next they'll
be pointing the finger at us in public.

Because to bottle-feed a baby is to be guilty of something. It's a crime against nature. Studies show that it is
rural women without college degrees who are the most
resistant to breastfeeding. They are eating "natural"
stuff all day long, so you would think that . . . But what
kind of "natural" are we talking about, in fact? Our
daily food, our clothes, cellphones, airplanes, UV
tanning, are these natural? Come on! We're constantly
bombarded with chemical products, so when I hear the
word *natural*, I get really annoyed. And another thing:
even if breastfeeding is "better" for the baby, what are
we trying to do, create centenarians? Life expectancy
has never been higher; do we have to start living
even longer? I remember the state of total decrepi-
tude my father was in when he reached the age of

ninety. I'm not sure I want to live that long myself. And I don't intend to give up smoking, either – that's all I have to say.

Breastfeeding is slavery. First of all, it's painful. And have you ever seen a nursing woman's breasts? Not attractive. They're scored with creases, there are milk clots on the nipples – they're disgusting! What's more, the poor mother is locked into being totally available to the nursing child, to whom she is constantly attached. Continually on duty, in a state of serfdom, she can't have even one little cocktail or a beer because alcohol is forbidden, or it will end up in her milk. I asked one friend of mine why the hell she was nursing, and she replied in a dry and contemptuous voice, "It's a personal choice." Maybe. But more and more, it's a collective obligation.

4.
You get to keep having fun

Having children is an unconditional and irrevocable commitment. Whether to have them is therefore the most nerve-wracking decision you'll make in your entire life. Sometimes just becoming aware of this can trigger a shock; Postpartum depression and marital crises are particularly modern diseases, the result of grieving the life you used to have. The amount of free time and spontaneity you once had is drastically reduced, and will keep on shrinking. You'll be living on somebody else's timetable now, the baby's, strictly laid out for you by the nanny, the daycare schedule, and the school calendar. Here are some of the personal freedoms you used to enjoy before you were saddled with the kid:

- Sleeping through the night (very rare during the first few months).
- Sleeping in all morning (difficult when the brat comes and jumps on your stomach at the crack of dawn).
- Deciding at the last minute to go to a movie.
- Staying out after midnight: you have to relieve the babysitter, and if you do stay out past midnight, you have to either drive her home or pay for her taxi.
- Going to a museum or an art show: the kid starts bawling after just five minutes.
- Travelling anywhere except to stupid destinations featuring beaches, the sea, or daycare.
- Going away any time other than school holidays (this applies to people with children from five right up to eighteen).
- Drinking before the kid's bedtime, because putting a child to bed when you are drunk just isn't done.
- Smoking in front of your kid: nowadays it's a crime against humanity.

5.
Rat race plus rugrats: No thanks!

Life with kids is life trivialized: you get up every day at the same time to take them to daycare or to kindergarten or to school, then you go to work, then in the evening you rush home to look after their bath, their homework, and their supper, and get them to bed. And that's it. Every day.*

Criminals are released on bail wearing an electronic security bracelet that allows the authorities to track them wherever they go. You, you won't need one. Your kid will be your ankle shackles. Your traceability is assured. In the old Soviet Union, the regime allowed certain privileged people to travel to the West, but their kids stayed behind the Iron Curtain – a good way of stopping defection. Find the kid, and you find the parent. Wanted by the police? Thanks to your child, they will have no trouble finding you. In the working-class Belleville district of Paris, illegal immigrants are grabbed at the school gate when they come to get their kids.

---

* Éliette Abécassis, in her novel *Un heureux événement* (A *Happy Event*), describes the hell of motherhood as "sleepless nights, lost liberty, the tyranny of the daily grind, house arrest."

There are husbands who vanish when they were supposed to be going out for cigarettes, prisoners who give their keepers the slip, old folks who wander off from their retirement homes. But parents who steal away from their kids without a fuss, that's rare. It's a good idea for a movie, but I doubt that it would ever get a subsidy from the National Cinema Centre.*

It's the always having to be there that makes having children so exhausting. When I had a full-time job at the same time as I had little kids, I calculated that I was working seventy hours a week. Forty hours at the office, thirty looking after my children. Three hours a night, five days a week playing mommy, plus seven hours on Saturday and the same on Sunday. Fortunately, I was able to take it a bit easy at work – otherwise I couldn't have done it.

For some time now, overburdened parents have found a solution to this: alternating care. The child spends a week with the father, then a week with the mother. It's a sort of half-time family. Of course, for this to work, the couple has to have already split up. But that's just a minor detail when measured against what they are escaping from: the hell of domestic

---

* Even less from the European Union. The EU gives preference – I'm doing this from memory – to projects with "humanitarian impact or projecting a positive image of humanity." Think about it. Pasolini or Fassbinder would never get a cent, naturally: they don't make children's films.

drudgery, each task more depressing than the last. Equality is the pay-off for the separated couple.

The naive will say, "Oh, but looking after children isn't work!" Seriously? Raising kids means sticking to schedules, doing chores. It is sweat, tears, and guaranteed tedium. In Austria, women can now calculate the amount of time they've devoted to child-raising when they negotiate their legal age of retirement. If looking after children were agreeable and rewarding, people would do it for free, but that is not the case. Nobody wants to look after *your* children without financial compensation (except, of course, your own parents, who will exact some form of payment eventually, which I'll get to later). The daycare worker, the teacher, the babysitter – they all get paid. Not very well, mind you: all the jobs connected to children are undervalued, and "child professionals" find themselves always less well paid than those who look after adults. Child psychologists: aren't they less respected than shrinks for adults? And schoolteachers are paid less than university professors. Why? Because they have undertaken a painful and unrewarding task. The child – what a dreary subject!

6.
You keep your friends

As is well known, love makes you stupid. The smitten man who talks about his sweetheart non-stop for hours, listing her wonderful qualities and quoting her *bons mots*, drives everyone crazy. It's the same with the bedazzled mother, marvelling at the wonder her body has produced, who bores her friends to tears with her excessive parental devotion. As the great playwright Georges Courteline said, "One of the most marked effects of the arrival of a child in a home is to render completely idiotic the wonderful parents who without it would have simply been imbeciles."

The insanity starts with the Sharing of the Birth. It's not just Evelyn and John who are involved in Anthony's arrival in the world but Anthony himself, who lets us all know that he has arrived *chez* Evelyn and John. The amazed daddy posts photos of the vapid family on the Internet, shows whoever wants to see – and many who do not – videos of the baby taking a bath or opening Christmas presents. He drives around with a "Baby on Board" sign on his car's rear window, a pious modern-day symbol that's about as useful for guaranteeing safety as a lucky charm. Every poor person who politely inquires, "How's the kid?" – the way we all say "How are you?" without really expecting an answer – is treated to an agonizingly detailed account of the lightning progress of his progeny. "Oscar is already using the potty." "Alice sleeps right through the night." "Noah built an incredibly realistic snowman." "Yesterday Ulysses said, 'Papa poo poo.'" "Jackson's passed second grade!"

There is simply nothing quite so narrow as the conversation of a man who is star-struck because he has successfully created a human being. And so when the child appears, the friends disappear. Soon the little darling starts answering the telephone, which means that it gets even harder to even reach the parents. Jules (or his sister Georgia) works up an ultra-efficient filtering system for all those calls that don't interest him, by hanging up immediately on any adult voice he doesn't recognize. In Nanni Moretti's film *Dear Diary* (*Caro Diario*), the disheartened hero ends up totally renouncing phone calls to his friends. Then there's the child's voice on its parents' answering machine, saying that they aren't there: this is a way of declaring to the childfree friend, "My kid matters more than anything else in the whole world."

In any case, there is really hardly any dialogue possible between a new parent and a childless person, even if a little shared commiseration ought to bring them closer together. The childfree person casts a gloomy eye upon the unattractive life of the parent ("The poor guy – between tantrums and diapers, he doesn't get a minute to himself!"), while the parent pities his friend's "solitary life" ("The poor guy – at his age, with no kids, how sad!"). The incomprehension is total, each side believing the other to have missed out on all the good things in life.

On my left, the spur-of-the-moment outings, erotic weekends, mornings in bed, trips with friends; on my right, Owen's chickenpox, Leo's cello lessons, the babysitter who didn't turn up, Maggie's homework, a daycare strike. Is this a fair contest? The reader can decide.

Have you ever been to visit new parents who are overwhelmed by their kids? It's pretty frightening. When you show up around eight o'clock, the kids are manifestly not yet in bed, tearing around the house screaming and yelling. A quiet chat among friends is impossible, with the gremlins running in and out, shouting, doing all kinds of stupid, attention-getting things, throwing toys on the appetizers. While the parents try to calm them down with long explanations that convince nobody ("Wow, it's ten o'clock, time you got into bed for a nice sleep that will make you feel so much better. . . ."), the guest is supposed to keep on smiling, hiding his exasperation. After an hour of this chaos, the guest is doing his best not to say, "Either they settle down, or I'm out of here." Then comes the bedtime ritual, and you can count on a good hour before the monsters actually go to sleep. The parents feel obliged to let the children know yet again that they are loved, even though they've been saying it all day long. Meanwhile, the poor guest is losing all patience, wondering why the hell he didn't go to the movies. . . . And when the evening is finally over, he heaves a relieved sigh and lights a cigarette (at last) in the street, to calm himself down: he certainly hasn't been able to smoke during the evening – it's very bad for the children.

Let's imagine that this fuming guest who has just left agrees to be part of a family weekend. That's when things become totally intolerable. The family bellowing at the table, kids yelling in the night, exasperated parents, the religious observation of afternoon naps – the whole weekend is a disaster. Worst of all, the guest always comes second to the children. It becomes clear the parents couldn't care less about his well-being. And he will have to put up with a multitude of vexations and annoyances – the baby's bedroom door left open all night so that it doesn't suffocate from the heat, the impossibility of doing this or that because it "upsets the children," and so on, and so on. Some day, when their children are grown up, the couple we are describing here (any resemblance to actual people is not coincidental) will find themselves all alone with no friends, in a bungalow in the suburbs, counting their retirement benefits. You have to wonder: is this the way people actually live . . . when they have children?

7.
You won't have to use that idiot language when talking to kids

There actually is a special language for talking to kids. Ever wanted to learn it? I shall explain the basics to you.

The French version of this language does not allow
the imperative, which is replaced by the indicative.
You don't say, "Camille, say goodbye and go to bed,"
but, "Camille, you're saying goodbye and you're going
up to bed." The most common phrase of all is, "You
are calming down." Or, "We're calming down," which
is repeated like a mantra – and is normally totally
ignored. If the imperative is ever actually used, it's
ineffective. "Sit down" (as opposed to "Let's sit down")
is repeated over and over again as a sort of refrain.
Usually you speak to kids in the present tense, the
future quietly being allowed to disappear: "Papa is
coming in a moment," "Tomorrow you are doing your
homework." And as for the past tense, there's only one
form – the present perfect: "Have you cleaned up your
room, Melissa?" With children, language resembles
a nursery rhyme.

We don't dumb things down any more with cute
words. No more "The little poopsie has cold tootsies" –
that's been banned. It retards the child's development.
She is supposed to leap directly into the real language,
that of grown-ups. And you have to speak to the child
about everything, no matter what. There's nothing
more ridiculous than these *mères de famille* who talk a
steady stream to their little two-week-old monkeys, who
don't understand a word. "Mama's going to change
your diaper, Kevin, you've done a nice big poo-poo.
Mama's going to change your diaper and then we're

going to see Grandma – you remember Grandma in the big house near the station?" This can go on for hours. Some even speak it in public. But you do have to be holding a diaper to do it properly.

When the children are a bit older, you can expect to hear parents saying sugared-over things like, "Cassandra, if you burn the cat's fur like that, he might die, and you really don't want him to die, now, do you?" – this, to the wretched little creature while she's trying to torture the neighbours' cat (which, fortunately, is capable of looking after itself). Certainly, there are no accompanying slaps or raised voices. You must operate by persuasion. "You have to explain it to them," preferably by going on your knees on the floor, so as to be at the child's level – otherwise she might feel looked down upon. The well-intentioned parent will work hard to devise forms of authority unknown when they themselves were young, forms designed to persuade rather than to produce obedience. Interesting that the same kind of thing is going on in business now, where authority has been replaced by dialogue, and dialogue by communication!

The child, for its part, returns tit for tat, treating the adult like an imbecile, speaking in a language that is in keeping with all this. Children's talk swarms with boring questions, such as "At the swimming pool when you relax, can you make yourself sink without moving?" or

"Would you like me to give you a very painful injection in the heart that'll turn you into a tree?" It took me some years to admit to my kids that I was not interested in replying. You're not supposed to do that. You can't say, "Shut up, I'm thinking about something important." The solution is simple: don't listen. My kids think I'm just distracted – which is not untrue. When they're yammering at me, I frequently find myself drifting off into pleasant mental spaces – the books I want to write, vacations on my own with a stranger on a dream island, or simply a night of Beaujolais with some girlfriends. In a word, childfree.

As the children get bigger, things get worse. Their vocabulary becomes sadly limited, their speech choppy and awkward, every sentence broken up with "Fuck!" feelingly uttered. Their use of the word *like* defies belief: "Like, I was talking on the phone . . ." or, "Like, I don't care?" And *go*, that's another one: "Like, she goes, I'm gonna kill myself, and, like, I go, Wait till tomorrow, I'm beat." And *cool*: "Like, too cool, I saw them and that was, like, awesome?" "It was like, whatever, they, like, throw you in with somebody? You deal, right?" If you met somebody at a dinner party or in a bar who talked like that – would you want to continue the conversation? Child-parent dialogue is insanity. Without relief.

8.
Open the nursery, close the bedroom

Get that image of kids as little angels out of your head: child-rearing is war. And that's not just a metaphor. More and more parents are actually getting beaten up by their kids. While you're waiting for her to get old enough for you to legitimately give her a smack, your little sweetie will have you repeating things like, "Stand up straight," "Don't put dirty napkins on the table," "Chew with your mouth closed," "Clean up your room," "Pick up your dirty things," "Do your homework." The child, testing her power over you, will deliberately harass you until you're right at the edge. If you are raising several of them, it's double or triple indemnity, especially in blended families, which are said to represent "modernity" for lack of a more meaningful word. For a woman, this means raising not only her own children but also at least one of someone else's. Why don't we have vacation resorts for them while we're at it?

The worst thing is that children do everything possible to prevent you from having fun. That is the child's hidden face. And believe me, he is going to prove very inventive in this area. Just when you're finally about to escape for a night out, he'll get sick. He'll stop you from celebrating your birthday with your friends. He detests it when you bring a stranger home to spend the night – male or female. As for actually dating, don't even think about it if you don't want to traumatize the little darling. Children have an uncanny sixth sense: they know precisely when to start screaming, just as you're getting intimate with your boyfriend or girlfriend – assuming they're sleeping in their own rooms. Many kids today share their parents' beds. Twelve per cent of American parents admit to spending the night with their baby.* I highly doubt those parents' sex lives are anything to speak of. Goodbye, caresses; hello, sadness.

What could be more intolerable for a child alone in bed than imagining his mother and father making love in theirs? It's unthinkable. Moreover, it is probably the origin of the myth Freud invented for his *Totem and Taboo*, the son killing his father because of the good life he is leading – the bastard, with all those women, it's a scandal, it's unacceptable!* Up until the '70s,

---

* According to a study by the National Institute of Child Health and Human Development, it's got to the point where more and more American parents are visiting sleep consultants to try to get their children used to sleeping alone.

* My reading of *Totem and Taboo* is not very orthodox, I have to confess. (The reader may be more used to the following reading: In *Totem and Taboo*, Freud explains that the murder of the father, followed by a cannibal feast, was meant not only to prevent incest but also to give birth to relationships based on man–woman exchanges. Furthermore, it also laid the foundations of all religions, which celebrate, symbolically, the murder and devouring of the father.)

parents paid their children back in kind by enforcing strict but reasonable sexual restrictions: no intercourse before marriage, no hanky-panky before evening prayers. The sex lives of young people, especially girls, were rigidly controlled. But after all, that was only fair – tit for tat. You keep me from living my life, I'll put some serious limits on your liberty. It's war.

Sexual repression was never just about fear of unwanted pregnancy. For almost the whole of the 19th century, parents and teachers joined together in their struggle against an atrocious scourge: child masturbation. It was said to undermine children's health and leave them exhausted. It's hard to understand today how jerking off scared society so much back then, but let's try an explanation all the same. This fear is related to an enduring and powerful principle: one is not good, but two is okay. Based on this same principle, cloning is to reproduction what masturbation is to sex. Have erotic pleasure alone? Make a baby out of only your own genes? They're the same scandal. But why are they scandalous? Because it is not advisable to do alone what you could (and should) be doing with another. What a great way to force someone into a couple, someone who, left to herself, might well evade the fundamental needs of society by refusing – horror! – to reproduce. What does this have to do with children? The soothing and protective language society uses on that subject is a thin disguise for the subtext: Forward, march!

Ever since the Raëlians announced their so-called cloned baby, in 2002, the press has been talking about the "violation of all the laws against experimenting on humans" and the "irreversible that will inevitably follow," the "abomination, the monstrosity of this assault on morality." Why is it so shocking that a baby would be its mother's clone? Let's be serious. We're all clones already, not of one of our parents but of our neighbours and colleagues. The line is no longer "Love one another" but "Be just like one another." It's like tomatoes or green peas or potatoes: everything has to be exactly the same size in order to fit in the little boxes.

9.
Kids are the death of desire

Not every child kills love, but most kill lust. The aesthetic assault on the woman's body transforms her for months into something resembling an overstuffed beast, which forces her to dress in sacklike clothing. You can go on for as long as you want about how a pregnant woman looks gorgeous and fulfilled – I don't buy it. When I was pregnant, I saw myself as ugly, with a huge growth pushing out from under my breasts. A number of comments from friends between the fruit and the cheese convinced me of one thing they don't talk about a whole lot in *Today's Parent* or *Parents Magazine*: maybe a lot of men find their pregnant wives or girlfriends to be lovely enough, but they don't seem to want to make love to them.

And so with pregnancy comes a long sexual winter. And that's not a case of "I have good news and bad news": this bad news will not be followed by good. No, the deprivation won't be over when the child arrives. You just don't feel much like making love after you've had an episiotomy. And even if you do, it's going to hurt – for weeks. You don't know about episiotomies? The dictionary tells us that an episiotomy is "an incision of the perineum, starting at the vulva, used during childbirth." In other words, the butchering of the most intimate part of your anatomy, ladies – one of the parts that allow you to come. According to the medical profession, the episiotomy is a benign procedure; it's also widespread, at least for those who escape the ravages of a Caesarean section, which is a real piece of surgery. Maybe the episiotomy is a lesser evil, so we should rejoice in this?

And you're not going to feel much like having sex between diaper changes and the midnight bottle when you've already slogged through three hours of housework after getting home from the office. Surrounded by fighting and bawling brats, you won't feel much like making love. Even less so if you're in a cramped apartment, with the kids all squeezed in one room right next to the two of you. Can you imagine yourself in a steamy movie, like Kim Basinger in 9½ *Weeks*, with a bunch of

kids in the next room? The temperature drops immediately by nine and a half degrees, even with the world's
sexiest actors. Bye-bye, eroticism.

10.
Kids are the death knell
of the couple

Hel-lo, little one; bye-bye, sex. This one really is not
solvable within the family. Desire hinges on spontaneity, on the unexpected, on the inventiveness of the
partners, and it's going to be reduced to almost nothing
when you have a kid, let alone more than one. You'll
be first and foremost "Daddy" or "Mommy." You'll no
longer exist in the first person. When you talk to the kid,
you'll say things like, "Mommy doesn't agree that you
should put snot on the picture, Elijah." After a few years,
you'll see, you'll become *only* "Daddy" and "Mommy."
And twenty or thirty years after that, you'll be simply
"Grandpa" and "Grandma."

So does putting the children first really toll the
couple's final knell? Most of the time, yes. When you
have children, you can no longer be a capricious young
thing having fun with her girlfriends or arousing her
lover. You are no longer the high-spirited young guy
living like a bohemian, not caring about the state of your
bank account at the end of the month. You may become
"Grandpa" and "Grandma," but not necessarily with

each other. Statistically, your chances of growing old together are pretty small: raising kids will have exhausted them. You won't have been able to hold on to enough for yourselves. He will see only the matron who looks after the house and the budget and the kids; you will see only an old man with disgusting love handles who tinkers around in his workshop on the weekend and occasionally cooks something. Cinderella is transformed into a maid, Prince Charming into a toad.

Watching other couples becoming parents and completely sinking into their roles, I naively believed that they had just allowed themselves to get trapped and that this would never happen to me. Wrong. It happened to me, too. I hardly ever look in the mirror any more, or wear high heels; I never take my contact lenses out of their case; I buy new clothes maybe once a year. My partner is above all the father of my children, and they're pretty much all we talk about. When a man speaks to me at a dinner party, it never occurs to me that he might be flirting; if it does happen, months will pass before it dawns on me.

The result: in larger French cities, one out of every two couples gets divorced or separated, especially young couples. More and more couples are breaking up when the children are still very small: statistically, around the firstborn's fourth birthday, or shortly after the second child's, if they are a bit slow. To have sex, or to have children? It's often the choice you'll have to make.

11.
To be or to do: Don't decide

For a long time, the newborn child was seen as an eating and defecating tube, a view that corresponded to 20th-century obstetricians' description of the child as "the necessary and inevitable product of the delivery room." But in under thirty years, this thing has been transformed into a precious object endowed with its own special essence. A lot of shrinks, among them some of the great ones, have done their utmost to make it clear that babies – children – are not just objects: they are *subjects*, whose individuality must be respected. Which is true enough, but hello, misunderstanding. Parents believe that their adorable child is a blessing and must be catered to as the sole focus of their own entire existence. The child must never want for anything. They fall all over themselves to meet every need, needs that didn't even exist yesterday. Happiness is found in satisfying those needs. Yes. Repeat after me: *Happiness*!

And so by *doing* (looking after their kids), parents compensate for their own loss of *being* (the basic state of being a parent). There is no simple answer to the question "What does it mean to be a parent?" Once upon a time, it was clear: the parents were just Mom and Dad. But these days more and more children enlist a third person in order to get born: the sperm donor who takes the place of a sterile husband; the ova donor who stands in for the sterile wife; the *mère porteuse*, the surrogate who allows another woman to become the *mère de famille* to a baby that she, the surrogate, has conceived with the other woman's husband. It now takes three bodies, not two, to make a child. Blended families are no different: the step-parent who raises his or her partner's children is contributing to the "creation" of the child.

So who is the actual parent? The woman who gives birth to a baby conceived by means of another woman's egg implanted in her own uterus and then fertilized by that woman's husband – is she "completely" this child's mother? The man whose girlfriend is impregnated by the sperm of an anonymous donor – is he "completely" the father?

It's all frightfully complicated. But what is clear is that the looser the definition of parenthood becomes, the more we throw ourselves into *being* parents: the child has become the focal point of the family. Everything and everyone revolves around him, and the orbiting adults come in an ever-greater variety of combinations. Fortunately, there is a guiding light: "To have children is to give love," says a journalist in *Parents*, a magazine devoted to comforting parents with an identity crisis. *L'amour toujours*.

How simple.

How reassuring.

12.
"The child is a sort of vicious, innately cruel dwarf" (Michel Houellebecq)

Our contemporary concept of the child was largely shaped by Jean-Jacques Rousseau. The 18th-century writer (who, by the way, unloaded his own children onto an orphanage) very sensibly celebrated the connection between the child and the savage: each lives in direct communion with the world, understanding reality, in a state of purity as yet unaltered by civilization.

Let me be serious for a moment. St. Augustine said, "The child's innocence is vested in the weakness of its limbs, not its will." Children are like dogs: if they were two or three times bigger, they would be ferocious beasts, your very worst enemies. A lot of little kids you see interviewed on TV admit their ambition to grow up so that they can get even with their teachers, beat up their friends, and even kill authority figures. It is the subject of the movie *Honey, I Blew Up the Kid*: a distraught scientist, after a lab accident, watches his two-year-old son grow several metres tall and spread terror throughout the neighbourhood.

Think back to your own childhood. Other kids would tease you, steal your lunch or your allowance, make fun of your clothes, which were never "in" enough. A kid thinks nothing of grabbing another kid's toys, humiliating him in public, even hitting him – and then going whining to the grown-ups that people are hurting him, because children love to complain. By their very nature they consider themselves always the victim, never responsible or guilty. Remember *Lord of the Flies?* This edifying book tells the story of a group of boys stranded on a desert island who end up killing each other. This is happening in the real world more and more. In late December 2006, a twelve-year-old student in Meaux was kicked to death by two of his eleven-year-old friends. A few months before that, a little Spanish girl, thirteen years old, was beaten so badly by three girls in her class that her right leg was broken in several places. Lord, forgive us our childhoods.

The child preys upon other children, but is also a major nuisance for adults. Travelling with little kids on the TGV is a real test of your nerves.* Kids are yelling, spewing soft drinks on the curtains, kicking the seats. You used to be able to retreat to the smoking car, but they took that away. I suggest that the railway company sell "no kids" tickets at a premium, for seats on special cars – an idea doomed to infamy on the politically correct scene, but commercially? A sure thing.

Even worse than a train trip is living beneath a family with kids in a badly soundproofed apartment:

---

* The train à grande vitesse is France's high-speed train system. (Ed.)

that is the Way of the Cross. They're yelling, scraping chairs over the floors, banging toys around to wake you up at the crack of dawn. I know some people who have simply had to move.

Similarly, living anywhere near a school is a synonym for trouble. Take a small example drawn from daily life, which is an unparalleled source of valuable information. This harmless little matter concerns problems caused by children on their way home from school. Some parents received the following letter: "For several months the neighbours of the Lycée Française have been complaining about the nuisance caused by the rudeness of some pupils, both on the public streets and in private buildings. It appears that groups of pupils leaving their classes are the cause of some unpleasantness, and certain others are guilty of incivilities such as throwing garbage around and other forms of carelessness in regard to both public and private goods."

Advice: when you get an apartment, find one near an old people's home, even if you have kids of your own. At least you won't be bugged by other people's brats.

13.
Kids are conformists

Nobody is more of a conformist than a child. It's normal. He apes the adults, the bigger kids, even those his own age he's jealous of. The child spends his child-life wanting to be somebody else in order to be popular. It's when he gets older that he realizes that growing up is not an end in itself . . . but then childhood is over – it's too late to make the best of it.

Always wanting to be somebody else, the child is never satisfied with himself. He's afraid they'll make fun of him, give him the finger, criticize his sweater or his backpack. So he does everything his classmates do: he wears the same shoes, uses the same notebooks, adopts the same slang. Childhood is a long neurosis, for it is a neurosis to live in conformity with what you believe others expect of you. And all too often the neurosis of childhood is never cured but evolves seamlessly into adult neurosis.

Kids detest being different; they hate it when their parents do anything that draws attention to them. My kids told me that it just wasn't acceptable for their classmates see them in our battered old Peugeot 205. They didn't want their dad picking them up at school in his patched old shorts. They had no idea that I work from home, writing my books or seeing my patients – the youngest told his friends for a long time, with considerable embarrassment, that "Mom doesn't have a job." Other kids' mothers leave the house the same time every day to go to an office: this shows that they have a real job, even if most of the time nobody knows what it is this Office Person actually does.

Not knowing exactly what a job consists of, a lot of children think it must be like school, complete with the obligatory stupid teachers. To kids, their parents' work has become a totally abstract idea. They will be well prepared, when they grow up, for useless and boring jobs. While children are still small, society expects from them a blind obedience to the rules and to discipline: daycare, school – these are just links in the immense chain of control over the bodies and souls that make up the world. There's really no essential difference between a daycare and the workplace: one looks after the child and the other after the grown-up. Children probably see this as normal. A heated room of their own, a timetable to follow, a cafeteria, some pals – a made-to-measure Lilliputian dream.

14.
Kids are a treasure, and will cost you one

Children cost a fortune. They are among the most expensive purchases the average consumer can make in a lifetime. In monetary terms alone, they cost more than a high-end luxury car, or a world cruise, or a two-room apartment in Paris. Even worse, the cost goes up as time goes by. Of course, the State lends a hand, through all kinds of subsidies (though watch out: you may not always qualify), bursaries, and college funding. But all this is nothing compared to what *you* are going to spend on the child yourself.

Children have to be fed, clothed, housed, and looked after, their school fees paid, and all of this can go on for eighteen to twenty-five years, sometimes even thirty. We know that it comes out to around 20 to 30 per cent of the average income, but curiously, despite the wealth of statisticians, including some whose job it is to examine the cost of children, we don't have exact figures. In fact, there is a conspiracy among "natalists" – those committed ideologues who are convinced that France needs babies to ensure a model country, a model that, as everybody knows, would wither irrevocably if it were to be deprived of its own offspring. Joël-Yves Le Bigot, president of the Children's Institute, has declared that "all those who really care about this country's democracy are telling themselves it is better that the French people do not really know how much it costs to raise children; otherwise they wouldn't have so many." Need I say more?

The secret to happy parenthood is obviously money, which will let you escape the constant servitude that goes with the job. Angelina Jolie, Sharon Stone, Madonna, Nicole Kidman, and Susan Sarandon are always depicted as fulfilled mothers; they never miss a chance to say that motherhood is the most important thing in their lives. The men are the same: paternity has revealed the profoundest depths to Johnny Depp, and all his life

Tom Cruise has just wanted to be a father. Having staff helps. A babysitter who sleeps over when the parents go out, a nanny who puts together meals when you are eating out with a girlfriend, a tutor to supervise the homework – that's the least you need to make parenthood tolerable.

But wake up: you are part of the lower echelon or middle class (more and more they're the same thing). You have to do all this stuff yourself. Whether you like it or not, you're going to have to learn (it's on-the-job-training, too) a whole list of jobs: nanny, tutor, cook, governess, police officer, chauffeur, nurse, psychologist, and job counsellor. And above all, actor – because children are the perfect audience for anybody who wants to play the part of a parent. . . . Well, up to their adolescence they are. That's a lot for one person to manage. Yet for all mothers' multidimensional flexibility, it's astonishing how little market value they have. Have you ever seen a company going out of its way to hire mothers who are more than forty-five years old? This proves that there is something really rotten in the sweet state of human resources.

15.
Kids are unbiased allies of capitalism

Consumption is the foundation of parenthood. You have to equip yourself with a fantastic catalogue of stuff if you're going to be a parent worthy of the name: a cradle, a playpen, a crib, a car seat, a high chair, a carriage, a folding stroller, a baby sling, diapers, clothes, bottle warmers, bottle sterilizers, ointments, creams, baby-wipes, a changing table. . . . Some of these things display a technological refinement that is as impressive as it is useless. Take the baby carriage. The very latest European models are called Vigour, Aéroport, Carrera, Graco, Evenflo, Peg Perego, are offered with six wheels or even eight, inflatable tires, disc brakes, rear parking brakes, ergonomic handlebars . . . and on and on. They are little miracles. But now they are twice as heavy, difficult to drag onto public transit, impossible to load onto a bike or a scooter. You'll need a car to lug it all around. Preferably a big one, with airbags for safety. Every little trip turns into moving day, a nightmare of bags and totes.

This is costly, of course, but it is only the beginning. The child eats and soils himself, so you'll need a washing machine and a dryer and a dishwasher. And you'll have to get a big supply of plastic diapers (six or seven a day for two or three years) – a genuine environmental disaster, since they aren't recyclable. The little fellow requires some space, so you'll have to buy a house, where he'll have his own room – hopefully he will then be a bit less of a nuisance. Then you'll have to dress him, and there is an infant style book that the most committed parents take care to follow (buying the best brands, of course). All kinds of articles in women's magazines, as well as a sort of *Vogue* for children, called *Milk*, will help you choose clothes as expensive as those for adults. The dear little thing will wear them for only three months, if ever, but who cares?

For every single thing the child consumer needs, the parents must become consumers as well. But it is the child that is the major target of experts. The newer something is, and the more tawdry, the more she likes it. While still a toddler, she'll be playing Game Boy, and she'll have her first computer by the time she's eight. Technology is no mystery to her. At twelve, she'll have to have an iPod if she's not going to get laughed out of the schoolyard. But that's still not enough. A multifunction digital camera's next. And a cellphone: according to a British study, two-thirds of kids aged six to thirteen have one. What do they do with it? According to one expert in child marketing (a thrilling profession, I am sure), "All kids want one, even if they seldom use it except for calling home." Calling home? Don't kids and parents already have more than enough time . . . *not* to speak to each other? And besides all that, kids have terrible taste: ugly shoes in colours inspired by the latest video game, clothes based on some idiotic TV series, trading cards for Pokémon or Warhammer or Yu-Gi-Oh! Welcome to the Kingdom of Ugliness.

All that stuff means wasted money, wasted time shopping for junk, thousands of hours of work spent trying to earn enough to pay for a house big enough to store it all in. Parents have to do all this because every kid's room is an Ali Baba's cave, with toys stacked up to the ceiling and an incredible mess of clothes, boxes that have never been opened, gadgets that are broken or obsolete or wonky. In the Land of Merchandise, the child is in its element. It's great for capitalism – always more things, always more crap you can't recycle, inter-changeable junk soon forgotten and endlessly replace-able. . . . That is exactly what the child wants. As long as there are kids, the absurd world we live in has a future. The human species doesn't necessarily have one, but that's another story.

16.
A brain teaser:
How to keep kids busy

A few years ago, the Brits gave us a humorous and very British masterpiece entitled *101 Uses for a Dead Cat*. 101 Uses for a Living Kid requires a lot more imagina-tion. In the old days, kids played in the street and in vacant lots, amusing each other. Now, those vacant lots are filled with cars . . . and with kidnappers, the great fear of today's parents, who see them lurking around every corner. The days of simply telling kids, "Go out and play," are over, unless it's to go play alone in a suburban backyard. And I can tell you that's not their favourite recreation.

So the kids are kept inside, like they are in Boris Vian's novel *Heartsnatcher*, the story of a mother so tormented by the thought that something might happen to her kids that she ends up putting them in a cage.

On the one hand, capitalism has used kids as lab rats to test their products; on the other, they've given us many things in return. The former was free; the latter we paid for: that's the way it goes. It begins with the TV, in front of which the kid lies motionless for hours of brainwashing. The kid doesn't think he's doing himself any harm, but the upper and middle classes worry because they think TV is going to make kids stupid (and adults brain-dead, but for them it's usually too late). Those classes tend to choose more sophisticated stuff (Game Boy, PlayStation . . .), which kids are crazy about, and which are no more intelligent but still have the virtue of keeping them occupied. Long live high-tech babysitting.

But what parents love most is working up a sweat to make sure their kids are occupied intelligently. Start when they're really young, just a few months old. Kids' swimming pools are great for this. The principle is, you soak them in tepid (and probably urine-laced) water from the age of four months on. This is now so much in vogue that in Paris kids are enrolled at a swimming pool before they're even born. What is it good for? I have no idea, but here's what it says on one of the websites devoted to this form of recreation: "The child learns to become more self-reliant, and this stimulating environment benefits its psychomotor development. For many children, the pool is their entry into the social environment. This early socialization improves the quality of their future relationships." *Self-reliance, development, socialization*: the key words for a successful education. And all this happens in just a few weeks. If your children are not going to a kids' pool, they'll never amount to anything in life – you can count on that.

Later on, you'll have to enrol your kids in a whole load of after-school activities, which usually means taking them there and going to pick them up afterward. Look at the horrifying schedule* of Antoine, age eleven. Monday, guitar, from 5:30 to 6:00 p.m., Tuesday, handball, from 5:15 to 6:30. Thursday, music lessons, from 6:00 to 7:30. Friday, more handball, from 5:30 to 6:30. Every other Saturday, children's orchestra rehearsal. This marathon use of time – is it really designed to keep the kids busy? Or is it for the parents, who must, of course, take them there and bring them home?

---

* *Le Monde*, September 7, 2005, "Choose extracurricular activites without overloading schedules", by Sylvie Kerviel.

"Intelligent" activities are those that improve the child's performance at school, indicating that the child will, later, be fit for the job market. Chess and music lessons belong to this category. Parents can also choose creative activities, like drawing, or theatre, which is very good for helping one feel at ease in public. Everything must contribute to the child's "fulfillment" – an endlessly repeated word: *épanouissement*, the key to "personal development," for which there are tested recipes that will always lead to happiness. As for sports, there the child will develop team spirit and a taste for competition, both very useful when she gets a job.

But watch out: be careful not to overbook your kid. Don't give him the kind of workload you might expect from a plant manager, say. After all, if a kid succeeds the way his parents hope, that's what he'll end up being anyway. He'll have got the idea early on: no "wasted" time, no empty hours spent just sitting and watching the rain come down. Give him a preview of the real thing, the life of the wage earner – because winners are busy all the time, but losers couldn't care less. Losers may nevertheless be the avant-garde of the modern age: some day, in a world where there isn't any more work and not much to care less about, everybody will be on holiday or on the short work week or maternity leave. When that day comes, the only people still working will be parents raising their kids.

17.
The parent's worst nightmares

Parenthood is the Way of the Cross, paved with a lot of stations. You don't have to put up with all of them, but you'd better recognize that some are unavoidable. Here are the worst:

Disneyworld, a town full of idiotic cartoons, dominated by underpaid people dressed up like ducks.

Water parks, where plastic-looking fish have been trained to jump to music in pools that stink of chlorine.

The grocery superstore, on a Saturday morning, when you have to stock the fridge for the week (with Raphael, who constantly yells, and Angelica, who wants to buy every stupid thing she lays her eyes on – heart-shaped lollipops, a tin of beans with some kind of hidden prize, a cake topped with a stuffed teddy bear, ultra-crispy chips, and so on and so on).

That wretched little park with a few scraps of green that is the only kind of urban playground left for kids. On weekends it's almost impossible to escape taking the kids there: they're like dogs – they go nuts if they can't get out. Parents sit and wait for the time to pass (it will take a while), and in the wintertime they freeze. They will have brought a newspaper or a book* in an

---

* Such as David Abiker's *le musée de l'homme* (Éditions Michalon, 2005), a work that deals very fairly with parental fatigue duty.

attempt to ignore the spectacle in front of them: sand flung into eyes, kids getting pushed around, scores being settled, flower beds being wrecked, racist jokes. . . . Nothing is better proof of the total failure of a fair and dignified human society.

The suburban bungalow with a little garden, bastion of the proliferation of the suburban family, described by the feminist Betty Friedan as "a comfortable concentration camp."

McDonald's, where you're served foul, greasy food in a cheap Formica environment where they give away trinkets as prizes. The kids' four-star restaurant is the parents' gulag. The only good side: it's over quickly.

Nature Game Parks, which perfectly illustrate the expression "Keep moving, there's nothing to see." What you can see, in fact, is tourists trapped in their cars.

Kids' movies, each one more insipid than the last. *Inspector Gadget, Finding Nemo,* the *Harry Potter* movies, *Babe, Lemony Snicket's A Series of Unfortunate Events, Pocahontas, Teenage Mutant Ninja Turtles III.* . . .

August vacations, as tedious as it gets – traffic jams, packed parking lots, crowded beaches, uncomfortable "suites" booked six months ahead at an outrageous price. And what about a kids' room or "club"? If not, maybe September will come quickly.

And above all, the pinnacle of abomination: Christmas. Armies of parents charge into the stores to buy even more toys – the newest, the noisiest, the trendiest. What for? To prove to themselves that they are good parents. It's a task as never-ending as it is expensive, buying yourself a clean conscience, especially since everyday life doesn't offer a lot of opportunities for that. Then you immortalize The Day with a digital camcorder, to capture the precise (and rare) instant when the kid, unwrapping presents under the tree, takes on an expression of delight tempered by idiocy. This requires precision and diplomacy because drowned in this celebration of useless and expensive junk, the kid is soon bored (he would probably have more fun down in the garden pulling the legs off a spider). This gift-opening ceremony has to be filmed in its entirety, year after year, so as not to miss a single nanosecond. Show the film in a loop, hours at a stretch: it's an apt metaphor for capitalism – always more Things, never more satisfaction.

18.
Don't be fooled by the "ideal child" illusion

Beautiful, poetic, ideal – that is our vision of the child. She embodies the dream of a lost golden age, which, like every golden age, never really existed. Films like Christophe Barratier's *The Chorus* (with 8.5 million paid admissions) or Stephen Daldry's *Billy Elliot* play on that theme and are in fact reactionary: their mass appeal lies in their nostalgia-inducing quality, both nostalgia for the past and nostalgia for a lost childhood. Since children always attract viewers, TV uses them as an excuse for the most vacuous programs conceivable. This includes the telethon in aid of children with genetic diseases (a veritable Yom Kippur of good feeling, starring Generosity itself), in which a titanic effort is made to collect the greatest possible amount of money in the shortest possible time. What wouldn't you do for sick kids? The result is obscene and profoundly stupid. But hey! It's for the kids.

Curiously, childhood has become an ideal that leads adults into illusory dreams. It is no longer children who dream of freedom and growing up, as Benoît Duteutre stresses in his book *The Little Girl and the Cigarette*, but rather adults who dream of childhood as a paradise that they will never again visit. Except on TV. What other explanation is there for reality shows like *Star Academy*, in which adults *voluntarily* go back to school, where they sleep in dormitories, learn to sing and dance, squabble, and then get publicly forgiven. Television shows just worship childhood, even when – or *especially* when – it's adults who write and act in them.

News programs (the "news" part is a misnomer) are also crazy about kids. They cover all kinds of sordid stuff: lost or murdered children regularly open the 6 o'clock news. Folks want it, it seems. In France, they adored little Gregory, an unsolved murder they talked non-stop about for months, maybe years. It was breath-taking suspense. It's as if nothing really happened in the world between the Gregory story, in 1986, and 1989, when the Berlin Wall came down. Fortunately, a few years later public opinion (or the journalists – it's hard to tell the chicken from the egg) got to sink its teeth into murders committed by Marc Dutroux, the filthy Belgian. Then there was the case of Andrea Yates, the Texas mother who drowned her five children in the bathtub. And the public was enthralled with the story of Natascha Kampusch, the little Austrian girl kidnapped at the age of ten and locked in a cellar for eight years. And they were righteously indignant over Véronique Courjault, the French woman whose two frozen children were discovered in her freezer in Seoul. They shivered over the story of the German who killed nine of his newborn children and hid their bodies in flowerpots. These modern Medeas bring out our morbid fascination. The wicked child murderer, the perverse killer of infants – they are monsters! But at home things are going just great, thanks: our kids are "fulfilled" and their parents "well balanced."

19.
Your kid will always disappoint you

The child is such sweet revenge. We procreate in order to exact revenge on a disappointing life. We are convinced we can save our child from the mistakes that we believe victimized us. Even worse mistakes can happen, of course, and to avoid them, mothers are driven to produce the ideal baby: it's a genuine mission. And it means work.

Countless families, convinced that their child is brighter than average, get her IQ measured at the age of four and start hunting down the perfect school that will let their future Einstein's brilliance emerge. How do you recognize the "gifted" child? Simple, his progenitors will tell you: "He (or she) is bored at school." Given the number of students who sit and watch flies zooming around the classroom, anyone would think every kid in school is a genius. Some parents may fret about the long commute for the very gifted from home to the special school and back, but in the end nothing is too good for them, *n'est-ce pas*? We'll do anything to succeed by proxy.

And yet the pediatrician D.W. Winnicott warns that what a child needs is a mother who is just "sufficiently good": anything more would be too much. The Good Mother mustn't take things too seriously, and this is where it gets difficult. If you can have a sense of humour about it all, you'll be able to tolerate the idea that your kid is not perfect. No kid is perfect, and you can be sure that the more parents dream of perfection, the more their child is going to let them down. Disappointing marks at school? So now we are among those slightly disillusioned parents who have to revise their idea of little darling's giftedness. The funniest thing is seeing those parents who at one time were amazed by their kid's capacity and are now having to confess (or at least pay lip service to) the fact that this one at the age of twenty, well, he didn't quite succeed at getting his high school diploma, and her, well, she's doing some kind of lower-level studies at the local college, or trade school. . . . Oh, the shame of it all, for a child who had the mark of a genius!

And then later, if the little darlings, instead of becoming self-reliant, adaptable, and responsible, turn out to be hopelessly immature, well, it's simply disgraceful. If they don't have a job and are condemned to perpetual free time (the curse of the poor), then nobody will ever ask for news of them. Now take it a step further and suppose that a child, however well raised in the most virtuous, the most stimulating, the most pluralist and charitable modernity, becomes anti-democratic, anti-European, anti-progressive! But of course that's not really possible in France, at least, since the polling stations are set up in schoolyards, and so by definition will contribute to the country's radiant future.

But worse still, supposing he or she becomes a terrorist. Heaven forbid! Such a well-integrated person? In such a successful model society? They could never dream of giving that up!

20.
The horror of becoming a *merdeuf*

Merdeuf is the popular current colloquialism for *mère de famille*, implying that, to be a *mère de famille* you are above all, well, a *mère de famille*. *Merdeuf*. She has a job, of course, but that is for financial reasons and also because as a way of life, being a *mère de famille* is not very fulfilling. Her own mother can testify to this. The *merdeuf's* mother spent her whole adulthood as a house-wife and devoted her life to her children, constantly reminding them that she had made serious sacrifices for them, had turned down opportunities that would have been very satisfying and financially rewarding, namely, a job. The majority of forty-year-olds of my generation were brought up by this kind of woman, who committed herself to housework and the raising of the children and was completely frustrated by the emptiness of her life. Chronic fatigue, loneliness, disappointment, overeating, obsession with her children. Often fat and spilling out of their disgraceful old clothes, our mothers were nags. The modern *merdeuf* has sworn to herself that she'll do better.

But nothing has really changed, because the *merdeuf's* main job is still the kids. The typical *merdeuf* has her kids' photo on her desk at work and another in her purse, and she shows them off at every opportunity. She doesn't work on Wednesdays* because that is the day that she organizes all their stuff, drives one to a birthday party, another to karate class. She's always nibbling a bit from the meals she's going to serve them, but she's also thinking about going on a diet, and drinks mineral water. She doesn't have a whole lot to talk about, since she spends most of her weekend looking after Lily, Matthew, and Jeremy. Whenever you try to draw her into conversation on topics of interest to non-parents, she starts going on about her son's performance at school, her daughter's artistic gifts, and the comparative virtues of the schools in the suburbs. In short, people are going to avoid her like the plague – except other *merdeufs*, who understand that the child is a sacrament which requires sacrifice, the giving of one's entire self.

She co-ordinates her time off with the school vacations, these being quite long in France: ten days around All Saints' Day, two weeks at Christmas, two weeks in February, two weeks at Easter, two months in the summer – nearly four months during which she will either have to sacrifice her own time off or else send the kids to their grandparents or to summer camp, both options that demand a miracle of organization.

---

* The education ministry in France recently (and controversially) declared that all schools will be closed on Wednesdays. (Ed.)

Fortunately, the thirty-five-hour week has allowed her to organize things so she can be mostly at home. This profligacy of school vacations has had quite an effect on the workplace in France, and it's no wonder foreigners think that nobody in this country ever actually does anything. Truth is, offices are practically empty during school vacations. It's next to impossible to schedule a meeting between Christmas and New Year's, during spring break, at Easter, in August, or around All Saints' Day. So what? Globalization will just have to wait.

21.
Parent above all?
No, thank you

Even if she runs a company, sells millions of records, or has a thrilling job, a woman is supposed to say, "The kids come first." Increasingly, men are also expected to be parentally correct. Do you think that the two prime presidential candidates in the 2007 presidential elections, Ségolène Royal and Nicolas Sarkozy, would admit that their political careers were their prime concern? But where do they spend the majority of their time? Not at home. Consider François Bayrou, also a candidate, whose family routine was described by *Le Monde*: "Six children, and his wife, Elizabeth, who mostly brought them up herself at Bordères while François was politicking in Paris."* No worries there. What a lovely portrait of the *père de famille*: perfectly tailored for the election campaign. Nicely played, François.

France has never had a childless president of the Republic. And in other countries there are not that many either; a *childfree* leader like German chancellor Angela Merkel is a remarkable exception. Having children is clearly a real electoral advantage, which candidates are all too eager to exploit, splashing their family photos all over the media. President Kennedy set the tone in the 1960s.

I often think of that image of him at his table in the White House while his son is playing under the desk. Kids sell – it's that simple. They're walking billboards that declare, "You can trust my mom or dad. Vote for them in full confidence. They have kids – they'll understand your problems."

Hard to imagine a public figure admitting, "My work comes first: dogs don't need babysitters." That would be a public relations gaffe, most likely a career-ending one. Mother first, professional second, woman third: that's the winning formula. Don't try to reverse the priorities – it won't fly. Model Adriana Karembeu

---

* R. Bacqué and P. Ridet, "François Bayrou et son double," *Le Monde*, March 21, 2007.

got a lot of grief when she said, honestly and sensibly, "Children scare me a little. I'm not sure I have what it takes, or that I wouldn't repeat the mistakes my own parents made."

Well, she was right. Every *merdeuf* is potentially a bad mother and feels guilty about that. The simple fact of having brought a child into the world, especially *on purpose*, is the source of a terrible guilt. "I created a human being: I am responsible for that" – what a cross to bear! Every mother is afraid of being a Mommy Dearest, so she can never do enough: she can never look after the kids as well as she should; she can never be available enough; she's a poor listener; there are never enough snacks in the house, or balanced meals. Never enough, given that her own mother and her feminist friends have all told her that she has to get out and work, leaving her caught between the Scylla of the home and the Charybdis of the office. She is guilty. Guilty of coming home tired from work, of not singing lullabies at night, of having a meltdown after ten hours of yelling and screaming kids; guilty of feeling relief when she ditches the kids at daycare in the morning; guilty of being delighted when they go off on a school trip. At times she may even beg her children's forgiveness for not knowing what a good mother really is, for coming off as the wicked stepmother in *Snow White* without really meaning to.

What does "wanting a child" really mean? Do we know what we want when we want a child? Are we seeking *its* well-being? Psychoanalysis teaches that nothing is more dangerous than wanting good things for someone else, since you're simply projecting your own needs onto the other, and one day you are going to make the other pay for that famous *good* that you were trying to impose. Wishing someone else good fortune at any cost is ultimately destructive, because no parent is ever wise enough to know what she really wants for the children. To Marie Bonaparte, who asked him for advice on raising her children, Sigmund Freud wisely replied, "Do whatever you like – whatever it is it will be bad."

In the past – and I mean only a few decades back – we put up with kids as a kind of unavoidable fate, which was far from perfect but at least had the benefit of absolving the parents of too much responsibility. Now, listen: I am not nostalgic for a time I never knew. But it is true that one is likely to take better care of, perhaps to *overcare* for, the child you really want. The spread of contraception may even have had some surprising effects: according to the authors of the book *Freakonomics*, it has reduced crime in New York. It seems that kids who were actually desired integrate socially better than kids who were not. It's not such a big leap from there to imagining that the pill and the

IUD have been sponsored by the System to ensure a more docile workforce.

22.
Keep the experts at bay

To bring up your child, you are going to need experts: social workers, pediatricians, speech therapists, psychologists – a veritable army of family medical professionals. How did our grandparents ever manage without them? Our society is obsessed with the physical, moral, and sexual problems of childhood. By the way, it's interesting that there seems to be a parallel here between the transfer of parental skills to professionals and management's expropriation, in modern business, of workers' technical skills. No connection? Don't kid yourself – one of the fundamental pillars of the world we live in is this: we are flooded with esoteric knowledge which only the self-styled experts can claim to make intelligible.

The modern family is under the surveillance of a therapeutic State that keeps it under constant control. These people are there to irritate you (which is true of everyone who claims to be helping you), and also to let you know that society is expecting something of you parents, and expecting a lot. So much, in fact, that you will have to go back to school in order to learn your job. That's no joke – Ségolène Royal has proposed it very seriously: "When incivilities are on the rise, we will need a system of putting parents through mandatory courses in child-rearing,"* she said.

And while you're on the waiting list, here are your duties, parents. It is appropriate that you have authority, of course, but also that you "dialogue" with the child. That you spend dozens of hours a week at it. And at the same time, both members of the couple need to have well-paid jobs, so that the child is not "smothered" with care, especially maternal care. (This is the case in France, at least – in Germany, the idea of the working mother is not so well regarded.) It is important you become moral alter egos, focused on the well-being of the child and on the child's respect for moral values. Be well balanced and responsible. Steady and instructive. Open-minded and ready to stimulate the child's curiosity. Be everything and its opposite all at once. The final goal? A child who is "structured" – that is to say, on a leash. The ideal is the conformist child who knows what the limits are: in other words, who has been rendered sufficiently obedient by its parents that others will be able to manage that child too.

They're a chatty bunch, this corps of experts.

---

* From a speech given by Ségolène Royal on May 31, 2006, in Bondy. www.lefigaro.fr.

Pediatricians, psychologists, educational scientists – they're all devoted to the problems of childhood, and their teachings are fed to parents through a huge number of popular parenting books, which, despite their narrow intellectual range, are welcomed by many publishers with open arms. It is quite a lucrative field. Taking the prize for stupidity, right at the top, would be 100 *Recipes for Boosting Your Child's Intelligence* (I omit the author's name for charitable reasons). Some of these works have become real bestsellers, such as those by the prolific William and Martha Sears et al. (*The Discipline Book, The Attachment Parenting Book, The Breastfeeding Book, The Successful Child* . . .), which have already dethroned the classics of Dr. Spock. Those poor confused *merdeufs*, they are all diligently studying these books looking for the recipes that will help them raise their children well. Physical and mental health are not matters for the mother's own judgment but must match the rather ill-defined image of what constitutes a good mother. And then if she starts wondering whether all of this good advice is getting her anywhere, she can always turn on the TV and watch *Super Nanny*. Millions of viewers watch this popular series, a show, the channel's website tells us, about "a nanny unlike other nannies, who restores order to families where authority has been eroded by indifference." Or, in plain language, practical methods for controlling those little darlings who have wrecked their parents' lives.*

These Gurus of the Family, these "specialists" in childhood, are very good at promoting new fads. Where have they all come from? Nobody knows. Some of them are pure fantasists. I remember when my daughter was born a dozen years ago, the big thing was to "diversify" the bottle. Have you ever tried making a weeks-old baby swallow a spoonful of boiled spinach, or orange juice, or beaten egg white? It is not possible, but in the mid-'90s you had to attempt it: your child's dietary balance was at stake. Headaches and nervous collapse were guaranteed. The tide turned a few years later when it was determined that too much diversification gave our dear little ones allergies. So they stopped telling parents to be nutritionally adventurous. And of course, there is a Way of Doing Everything: putting the child to bed, changing the diapers, what kind of stroller to use. Kid science is by no means perfect yet, and our experts do seem to flounder a bit, despite the airs they put on. Should we throw out the baby with the bath water? It's up to you.

---

* The series is also a wonderful antidote: watching it once is equivalent to six months' pondering whether you really want to have a child.

23.
The family: A horror

Kindness, affection, spontaneity – these are the sheltering roles of the family, a comforting refuge from a public environment that is increasingly dominated by the impersonal mechanisms of the marketplace. Family life – idealized, magnified, a refuge of authenticity where people are allowed to "be themselves" – is clearly an *image d'Épinal.**

Well, tear up the postcard. The contemporary family is, in fact, an inward-looking prison, based entirely on the child. The family means scoldings under the Christmas tree, painful and unasked-for "moments of truth" with your mother-in-law, resentment that has been simmering for generations, shameful family secrets that nobody dares name but that are a burden to all. The majority of murders and of acts of pedophilia occur within the family. That should be food for thought. Every family is an inescapable nest of vipers.

Bonjour, neurosis; hello, psychosis. Child–parent relationships are not a piece of cake. It's not just love; it's also hatred, resentment, jealousy – all those feelings

---

* Sentimental 18th-century-style woodcuts and prints, still popularly sold in the northeastern district of Épinal, these depict a lyrical rural family lifestyle and are also widely available on postcards. (Ed.)

we don't talk about because it's just not done. You don't have to look too far to find them. Psychoanalysis has been very clear on this issue. Freud explained that the little boy wants to kill his father so that he can go to bed with his mother, and what could be sweeter or more endearing? Winnicott gave seventeen reasons why a mother might detest her baby: he is a danger to her body, he disrupts her private life, he hurts her breasts, he treats her like an idiot, he makes her follow his rules, he frustrates her . . . not exactly a rosy picture of maternity. If you have kids, you're going to have to deal with all these contradictions. A lot of people suppress them, which might just be the secret to idyllic parenthood. Is that better for the children? Not necessarily, because whatever happens along the genealogical trail, sooner or later somebody is going to have to pay the piper.*

But back to your family. With a kid, you're going to have a lot on your shoulders. Ironic, isn't it, because wasn't the kid supposed to be your way of paying your debt to the parents who gave you *your* life? You might think that you've gotten even now, but, no, it's not that simple. Parents and in-laws will be there to explain to you the art of child-raising and to drown you in ridiculous and unsolicited advice. And that will be nothing

---

* That is what psychoanalysis is good for: it lets other people pay the bill. Yes, it is costly.

compared to the veiled reproaches, the unspoken con-
demnations, and the endless little lessons whose
message is quite simple: you are an inadequate parent;
you don't know how to do it; your child is not fulfilled.
Little Jules wets the bed sometimes? Alexander has
eczema? Isabelle hates her math teacher? It's all your
fault. You moved in the middle of the school year; you
work too much (or not enough); you pay more attention to Isabelle than to Alexander – or the reverse. It's
because when you were a kid you were jealous of your
brother, or asthmatic, or in love with your sister, or a
stamp collector.

Psycho-talk is a big deal in families, where the
merdeuf wields it like an elephant in wooden shoes,
boasting of the Dolto she has in her library (but hasn't
really digested yet).* The *merdeuf* flings around an
oversimplified psychojargon like a kind of familial
Esperanto: "He's going through his Oedipus" (as if she
were saying, "His teeth are coming in"), meaning that
he is in love with his mother, and of course she is
delighted to have a little admirer in her pocket. "He
has a castrating mother," naturally, applies only to
other kids, who have terrible mothers, never to her
own child. "He's going through the anal stage" could

---

* Françoise Dolto, 1908–1988, famous child psychoanalyst and author. (Ed.)

translate as "He plays with his turds, which is disgusting, but normal."

The worst thing is that you are going to be trapped. Your family's or your partner's being an often-generous source of free babysitting, you are going to accept, with your mouth shut (yes, believe me), their *diktats*, blatherings, lessons, and double-barrelled psychological arguments. You will feel less guilty parking the baby with family than with a babysitter: that vile mercenary can of course be useful sometimes, but she doesn't love the kids – she's just paid help. In any case, listen: getting away from the kids for a few hours or a few days is a pleasure worth paying for. But it is not always payment in money that costs the most.

24.
Don't revert to childhood

The child is the high priest of taste. The Young Look is all the rage. A lot of mothers try to dress like their adolescent daughters – a short little sweater, navel showing. Kid's taste is becoming almost everybody's style. It used to be that young girls imitated their mothers and dressed up like ladies; now women copy their daughters and dress like waifs. Exit the sexy and mysterious dame incarnated by movie stars in the old days; it makes you wonder why the big designers go to such lengths to dress real women, when women don't even want to *be* women any more. Look how young the models are getting! Only childhood is really sexy, not adulthood. Tomorrow's fashion models will be preteens because in the new semantic world, childhood has shortened: it's over far sooner than before, at around age ten. After that, watch out – you're running out of time.

All that stuff designed for kids is destined for cult-hood, like the Kinder Surprise toys that have become trendy among adults and are apparently already showing up in museums: puzzles, figurines, miniature cars, rideable robots, things with valves and knobs. . . . Fine, it's art, right; but more than anything it is a market, around which hover experts, collectors, gallery owners, investors, and even frauds.*

Adults adore products intended for children and have taken over quite a few for their own purposes: kids' furniture, toy cars, miniature everything – pocket vacuum cleaners, mini beauty products, baby wine cellars, baby beer barrels, Heineken XXS. If it's tiny, it's cute. What is the adult's dream? To live a minia-ture life in a little kid's room. And what's the advan-tage? When you treat yourself like a child, you don't have to look after your own kids – because you won't have any.

---

* Funny profession, no? Imagine a business card that says "Fabricators of Fake Kinder Surprises." It's funnier than a racist joke.

Children are the new tastemakers, even for books. In France, the *Unpublished Stories of Father Christmas* was a lightning success: 650,000 copies of volume 1 sold when it came out in 2004. One of the biggest sellers in the world is *Harry Potter*, and if you want to be in the loop, you have to have read the latest instalment and be prepared to discuss it knowledgeably should it come up in conversation. If you haven't read it, then you've just been left behind. All the same, what has come to be known as the "Harry Potter phenomenon" (learnedly analyzed by shrinks, sociologists, and philosophers) at least doesn't pretend to be more than it really is: a kids' book.

Getting in on the action, bookstores now have entire walls of "young adult literature." And you can bet on there being more and more of it. Why bother reading books that are difficult? "Young adult literature" is a great example of an oxymoron, meaning a combination of contradictory words. I don't think Kafka, Shakespeare, Proust, or Cervantes ever wrote books for under-twelves.

The success of the "young adult" market has spawned imitators. There's a growing tide of literature for adults that resembles . . . literature for children. Literature-for-children-meant-for-adults is riddled with gems like *Antéchrista,* by Amélie Northcomb, which tells the story of two very different girls, close friends who are jealous of each other, and *Oscar and the Lady in Pink,* by Eric-Emmanuel Schmitt, in

which a very sick child meets a mysterious lady –
appropriate for ten-year-olds, maybe even eight-year-
olds in the latter case. This kind of dumbed-down stuff
has, nevertheless, a very useful social function: it gives
adults who do not read the illusion of having nonetheless scrounged a few crumbs of so-called culture.
Alexandre Jardin, with *The Zebra*, went one better: here
was a book that spoke to the child slumbering within
every adult. But it was in his *La révolte des coloriés*
that he really outdid himself, celebrating the child
king as a stellar novelty, the spontaneity of youth, the
natural lack of inhibition, the innocence. It is an
appeal to us to awaken within ourselves the "most
authentic elements" supposedly crushed by the "civilization of grown-ups."

Welcome, puerility!

25.
It takes real courage
to keep saying,
"Me first"

The family is a group egoism that repudiates the indi-
vidual. It is not, as is sometimes said, the product of individualism gone wrong. The evolution of the last few
centuries is often seen as the triumph of personal liberty
over social constraints, among them the family. But

what happens to individualism when a couple's total reserves of energy are given over to the children? The development of contemporary mores demonstrates, on the contrary, the prodigious explosion of familial sentiment. It is the family that has won out over social relationships, friends, neighbours. The family is Queen. This is not a good sign; it is the sign of a step backward for personal identity, as the media would say. The historian Philippe Ariès puts it like this: "Family feelings, feelings of class, and perhaps in some cases of race are manifestations of the same intolerance of diversity, of the same need for uniformity." In that case, could family be the basic building block of the National Front?*

We live in a society of ants, where working and reproducing represent the ultimate objective of the human experience. Work is the opiate of the people; will children be their consolation? A society where life consists of earning a living and raising your kids is a society with no future, since it has no dreams. Having a child is the best possible way to avoid asking what the meaning of life is, as everything revolves around that child, who is a marvellous substitute for the existential quest. "My son, my battle," as Daniel Balavoine sings. That's all very nice, but if that is your only battle, your life doesn't mean very much. The philosopher Alexandre Kojève

---

* The extreme right-wing party led by Jean-Marie Le Pen. (Ed.)

said "the animal defines itself by exhausting its existential possibilities in procreation." A lot of today's parents are not far away from that animal state.

To respond to the question of the meaning of life by simply reproducing yourself is to shift the question to the next generation. To not respond at all, or to not even try, isn't that the worst kind of cowardice? Isn't that a pretty heavy burden to put on the children? The sight of their defeated parents just dropping the ball is not the best example to set our dear little ones, either. One day soon the children won't hesitate to sit in judgment on their parents, and their verdict will not be very lenient, especially if those parents have been living a stupid life. A stupid life means being a servile little worker whose big concern is, for lack of anything better, developing his spiritual life; feeling his emotions more profoundly, perhaps delving into Eastern wisdom; going on hikes or taking up running in order to "feel better in his skin"; learning how to relate more "authentically" to other people; "overcoming his fear of pleasure."

Fortunately, citizens, you can sleep peacefully. Order has been established. Today's young people are a lot less defiant than those of 1968.* No way are they going to

---

* In May 1968 there was a month-long period of left-wing protests and a general strike that are thought to have eventually led to the collapse of the de Gaulle government. (Ed.)

be out in the streets protesting that they've been handed a load of shit, demanding answers, and upsetting the established order to get revenge. They are far too busy just trying to . . . fit into society.

26.
Kids signal the end of your youthful dreams

For tens of centuries, powerful pressure has been put on couples to stay united for the sake of the children they've made. It was considered appropriate that both members of the couple renounce their personal ambitions in order to stay together and bring up the kids. But nowadays, the theatrical "I have sacrificed myself for you" seems a bit outdated; many parents have adopted a line more in vogue with the times: "I have given up my dearest hopes for you, so that you will be happy. Fulfilled. So that you will have an excellent education. So that you can do graduate studies." The words have changed, but the hypocrisy is just the same. People who have no children are sometimes astonished by the amount of sacrifice made for kids who never asked for anything, and the answer they get is, "You could never understand: you don't have kids."

To paraphrase Céline about love, infinity, and poodles, the child is immortality at the level of a sheep. No, the child is not the adult's future. That is another lie society created to keep us quiet, and it goes like this: Your children will succeed where you failed; we will give them the means through education and social advancement; it's guaranteed in the contract. Paradise is for tomorrow, not today. Happiness is for your kids, not for you. While you wait for the great tomorrow that is winging toward your progeny, just keep quiet. One "My child may have this one day" is worth far more than any "I want this, here and now."

Isn't it?

Well, that's debatable.

You will often hear parents who have spoiled their own lives in the name of their kids say something like, "What else could I do – I have children to raise!"

"I can't quit a job I hate because I have kids"? What an excuse! "I haven't been able to pursue my own dreams – I had to feed the kids." What an awful thing to say, no? Before, in my parents' time, my mother said: "If I can't leave your father, it's for your sake." I realized that the real motive was that she would rather stay home and drive my father crazy and be driven crazy by him. There are those who would rather be unhappy together than happy on their own. That's the way it is.

In reality, children are often used as an excuse for giving up on life without even trying. The moral of the story is, when you do not do what you really want to do, there is no excuse. Not work, not the family, not your country.

27.
You can't stop yourself from wanting your kids to be happy

The happiness we want for children, that we promise them, is an odd thing. First of all, none of us knows what happiness is. Is it material well-being? Social success? Boozing and sleeping around? It's up to each of us to answer as best we can because nobody really knows. Happiness appears at the time of the American and French revolutions, and is even written as a right into the U.S. constitution. "Happiness, a new idea for Europe," Saint-Just said. Well, the truth is that it is a product of democracy and of the mass production of Ways of Life, where every person feels they have a right to a piece of the cake. To use the language of the futur- ologists, in an uncertain world it is normal to live in the present and gaze at your navel – at least that is what Michel Onfray * advises his many readers.

The growth of the importance of the word *happiness* is the result of centuries of progress, because we have always believed that tomorrow will be better than today. But promising a child happiness today is an act of bad faith. I'm not going to recite you a little verse on

---

* Elitist French philosopher, atheist, and writer on psychoanalysis. (Ed.)

the future of the planet, but there is not much there to be cheerful about. A hole in the ozone layer, global warming, overexploited forests and fisheries – that's what we are facing. And especially you, future generations, because you're going to have to pay for it. It's a pretty crappy baton they passed you; do your best: say, "Thanks very much." Your parents did what they could to make you happy. They certainly didn't try to change the world – they were too busy changing your diapers.

Parents struggle like mad for the happiness of their children. *Hap-pee!* In fact, parents don't promise their kids happiness: they demand it of them. "Be happy!" is a fierce and obscene injunction, coming from the superego Freud wrote about, that gives orders and at the same time tells you to play. Playing – that is suspect from the start; in a capitalist system, freedom always leads to the same end: the universal obligation to enjoy yourself and to give yourself to enjoyment. "Profit from life; play, my son" – that's a command with a built-in trap. Because at the same time, the parent is saying to the child, "Don't do this; don't do that; try to please your parents." If someone is trying to persuade you that all they want is your well-being, watch out, because the same person will inevitably feel justified in preaching at you, giving you advice, trying to make you do things you don't want to do. Besides, that kind of training is a mission eternally doomed to failure, because wanting the welfare or happiness of someone else is a sure path to devastation. Happiness? No thanks, no way, not for me.

28.
You can't get away from your kids

So what do you do with children? Everybody adores them, but nobody really wants them around. Spend years in the house looking after kids? You must know that this is death by boredom. Unlike in Scandinavia, there is no structure in most countries to encourage the *merdeuf* to take the kids with her to a restaurant or the movies. So she lives a monastic life, measured out in diapers, baths, and bottles. Looking after children soon proves to be more tiring than going to your job. The smart thing to do, if you can, is to find your way back to the job you left behind and pretend to be working. At least then you can spend the day quietly in your chair, head for the gym from noon to two, relax during coffee breaks, do your e-mailing, phone your friends for a couple of hours without being distracted. I would bet that's why so many women go back to work after they've had kids, to the point that it's the norm these days. I am focusing on women here because in our world it is still the woman who takes on the bulk of child-raising. Men, through either cleverness or laziness, always manage to get out of it.

All right, go to work then, but the children are still going to need looking after. How do you accommodate your kids to your schedule? Live-in help costs a lot. Problems pile up. You can't just stow the kids away somewhere. All the daycares, nursery schools, and kindergartens seem to announce that they're full on the very day you're finally ready to farm your kids out to professionals. So you need to plan well in advance: you will soon see that there are always more applicants than places – that's the iron law of the childcare world. It was already like that when I was little, but back then you could blame it on the baby boom; today it is "structural." And that goes for booking a spot in a daycare, let alone that ski holiday for your teenagers organized by the social committee at your office. There is really no place reserved for adults (which explains why anyone who manages to get one holds on to it for dear life). There's no place for tramps any more, either: all the public benches have been removed, probably not by chance. Keep moving, get out, look somewhere else. Seventy per cent of kids under three are looked after at home, mostly by their mothers.

So how do you get a spot in a daycare? In France, you have to stake out City Hall and fill out those very detailed (even intrusive) questionnaires: "How much do you earn? And your husband? You're not married? What level of education have you reached? Profession? Normal work hours? Do you own or rent? How many rooms are there in your apartment? How many people are living there? Any other family in the neighbourhood? Any health problems?" And that is without even looking at the esoteric questions about the "familial coefficient," the AIL, and the AJPE.* It is a real police interrogation. Well, what would you not endure in order to get rid of that eight-to-six burden?

Then, at the next step, when they reach school-age, the problems continue. You're required to send the kids to school, but getting them there is not easy. As at the daycare: there is a shortage of places, since "our classes are all full," "you are on the waiting list" (and clearly they're doing you a favour if they take you) – especially if you want a place in a high-quality school, or even in the least bad school in the area. In some districts politely referred to as "mixed" (lots of poor people, subsidized housing, ZEP),† parents have to choose between being good parents and being good citizens. They usually choose the first. Since it became impossible in France to choose what school our children go to, we have to jump through hoops if we want to have at least some choice – without appearing to do

---

* *Amis de l'instruction laïque* and *Allocations pour jeunes enfants*, both related to educational grants.

† *Zone d'education preferée* (Priority Education Zone), a system of subsidized schools in France. (Ed.)

so and without getting caught. So we need patience, dexterity, discretion, several trips to the Education Authority offices, sometimes a fake address, and a white lie or two to avoid the school where none of our neighbours want to send *their* kids. Yes, school is a kind of sorting machine, a formidable device for handing out social privilege and reinforcing class division, all the while hypocritically preaching equality.

Liberty, Equality, Fraternity . . . as long as you keep your place. Republican elitism – that's another nice oxymoron: there are the elitist schools on one side, and the "republican" schools on the other (which will accept anyone), but they don't accept the same students.

Into your kennel, kid – but not just any kennel.

29.
Get used to it:
School is a boot camp

Your children are going to spend the most important part of their young lives in school. This will help "socialize" them, their parents will say, meaning that it is good for them because even if they don't learn anything, they will be playing with their friends. However, school is not actually a place of open friendships and free expression. *Au contraire*: this is the kingdom of social control. After kids turn six, when nursery school and kindergarten are finished and the serious stuff starts, it is no laughing matter. It was at the end of the 17th century that what must be referred to as a "disciplinary regime" was established. Like lunatics, the poor, and prostitutes, children – who up to then had always been around adults – had to submit to a process of confinement. This quarantine was known as the "school," the "college," or the "lyceum."

A school is a place for discipline and indoctrination. It is designed for the average person, neither too bright nor too stupid, and those who conform to this model thrive. They learn to read in the year they are supposed to learn to read, not the year after. They put up with stupid assignments and never ask why. School is all about norms. It serves to format people for work, for the kind of routine that requires no special technical or intellectual competence. Industrial society needs people who have been stupefied, who are resigned to carrying out meaningless tasks and to never seeking any kind of satisfaction except in their free time. School is a wonderful waiting room.

The teacher reigns here, especially the female teacher, who is usually someone who disliked school when she was small; otherwise she would have done brilliant work and sought a more interesting and better-paid career. Your average school is a sour place, based on the stunted language of the teachers colleges, where they'll call a ball a "bouncing frame of reference" and a student "the learning one." These people use such

incomprehensible phrases as "the didactic triangle."
They are very quick to sense deviation, and orient
their students at all costs toward an army of speech
therapists and psychologists, thinking that they can
thus unload at least part of their workload. It is these
people with whom parents have to work out a non-
aggression pact – and that is not always easy.

One has to suppose that kids get pretty confused.
School seems to totally contradict the family discourse
based on "fulfillment." Whatever work the parents
don't complete will be up to the school and society at
large to look after. At school they don't want individuals; if your kid does not conform to the norm, it will be
up to you to straighten him out before they expel him.
I was put in my place by a teacher in a playground,
between a bust of Marianne and a heap of wooden
benches. It was all my fault if my child wasn't interested
in the curriculum, if he fought in the schoolyard, if he
left stuff at home. I was doing a bad job of parenting. It
felt like being in front of an examining magistrate.
There I was, mute, having to look contrite – I was terri-
fied my kid would be expelled. I was scared that, in the
middle of a crisis and in the middle of term, I would
have to find a private school that would be willing to
take him. It's hard, hard, to be the parent of a student –
especially of an "atypical" student, meaning one who
doesn't want to just fit in the box. Of which, it seems,
there are a growing number.

If the school doesn't manage to keep a kid in step, then the community takes over – in repressive mode this time. In 2005, Nikolas Sarkozy, then Minister of the Interior, put in his draft law on preventing delinquency the principle of "early identification of behaviour problems" among young children, problems of a kind that might lead to juvenile delinquency. Which means what? That within every non-normal (disturbed) child there sleeps a potential delinquent? And that society has a duty to clean up the problem at its source? Hello, security paranoia. . . . These ravings were based on a report from the National Institute for Health and Medical Research: long live science, the strongest ally of universal policing. Thanks to a petition entitled "No Dead End for Kids under Three" and the condemnation of the National Consultative Committee on Ethics, the draft law was thrown in the garbage can. But the tone had been set.

Permissive? France? Come on! The talk deploring this so-called permissiveness and the damage caused by the events of May 1968* doesn't hold up. It's the other way around: it is the lack of play and of flexibility and even of disorder that has rendered this society so smothering. People who don't fit the slots they were intended for are first put to one side, then penalized, then simply left to their own fate. That is what certain suburbs are

* See page 83.

all about, wild, disconnected. Or else shut your trap, as the song of the same title says,* just don't show your dirty face. Long live the French approach to integration, which has succeeded in disintegrating everyone who is not integrated.

30.
"Raise" a child . . .
but toward what?

Kids start bringing work home from school at the age of six – work they have absolutely no interest in doing, and understandably so. Grammar exercises written in pedagogical jargon, dreadful poems to be memorized – all contributing another layer of forced labour to the already overloaded parents' schedule. On top of that, everything that the kid has not understood at school now has to be explained at home. And the homework? Guess who gets stuck with it. It's usually the *merdeuf*. Let's hope that somewhere inside her there sleeps a frustrated classroom teacher because she is going to spend hours a week on this, until the kid becomes "autonomous" – which can take a long time. Sometimes the *merdeuf* is so exasperated by the kid's crankiness that she ends up doing the homework herself. It's a lot faster.

---

* Fatal Gazouka, *"Fous ta gueule,"* 2007. (Ed.)

Some evenings it would take me an hour and a half to get through that homework. And yet my children were educated in a public school (but you can call it "School for the Poor"), where, if what I hear is true, the teaching staff is less demanding than those in the very choice schools in nice districts. Helping them with their homework for all those years was unspeakably tedious. I have to say that when I was a kid, I detested school. Explaining things bores me, and I hate to have to repeat things. And with my own kids I had the impression that I was going through all those hateful lessons all over again, until one day, at the end of my tether, I finally let go and said to them, "Kids, do it yourselves, and whatever happens, happens!"

Their marks ended up just as mediocre as they had always been, but at least I was freed from having to wade through that desiccated dust of drudgery.

What makes the homework load even more of a scandal is that written homework isn't even supposed to be assigned in primary school, but the teachers seem to ignore this, probably to make themselves feel important. Furthermore, it's clear that homework is a contributing factor to current social and cultural fragmentation, since kids with a parent at home or with someone paid to help them are the only ones who will ever get it all done. Why do parents put up with this nightmare? Because they think it will be good for the kids – they'll be learning things that will be a valuable resource later on. At first I naively supposed that there was a small minority of knowledge *revanchistes** who were disheartened at having to be tutors every day. It was only after some years that I realized that everyone was infected with this virus of Grandpa's "good old methods": debates over learning methods, the return to school uniforms, sermonizing about work and effort, disputes over single-sex education. One day they'll want to go back to quill pens and whacking hands with rulers.

But school is not enough to put the child on the high road to the light of learning. Every self-respecting middle-class parent thinks that children have to read. They agonize about it: "How can I get the kid to read?" It's an important challenge: the dear little one's personal development depends on it, as does the growth of her intelligence and the flight of her imagination.

You can hear these typical chauvinists, totally taken in by all this, hardly reading a book a year themselves (and you should see *what* books), pronouncing on the importance of reading. They repeat to their kids the same mantra that we always got, and that no longer

---

* Members of a movement in France after World War I, who promoted revenge against Germany primarily in the form of the recovery of lost territory.(Ed.)

applies in a world where plumbers earn more than doctors or lawyers: "If you do well at school, then you're sure to get a good job later."

As a matter of fact, this is a complete misunderstanding, because reading is success's worst enemy. Children who read all the time turn into total flakes. When I was a kid, nothing else interested me, not school, not music, not hikes, not holidays. The result: I became completely asocial and incapable of teamwork. So does a real passion for reading in fact make you useless to your fellow humans? Well, I exaggerate. A bit. Sometimes kids who really love reading become the Auxiliary Troops of Intelligence, culture's casual labour – publishers' interns, bookstore clerks, underpaid and ill-regarded freelance journalists. In any case, they'll be overeducated for any jobs available in the marketplace. Eternally embittered, they'll see business meetings as a form of torture, taking on a project as overwhelmingly tiresome, meeting management for a job evaluation as the clash of two different worlds. Now numerous, these misfits are doomed to extinction because young people are reading less and less, especially those who graduate from the prestigious institutions, famous big schools, and the like. So let's get on with it – the nation's élite just has to produce books and culture. Get thee behind me, Satan!

31.
Avoid benevolent neutrality like the plague

A baby, as they keep driving into us, is really a person. It's the shrinks that put that idea in our heads. Freud was actually the first, in his practice, to let a child (Little Hans) have its say. He was followed by Dolto, and Winnicott too. And this wasn't some cozy little scene, because when these pioneers started really listening to children, they heard some pretty disturbing things. But a lot of educators nowadays think that communicating with children has only one purpose: helping them integrate into the larger world – making sure they feel good, that they express themselves. In short, the language that they use and that they provoke is purely decorative – it has no effect, it serves no purpose. It is about as useful as an office memo: you trade junk back and forth, but you do it with conviction.

Communicating with children does, of course, have a purpose: to make kids do what they're told. This is tough because parents don't give their kids orders any more, resorting to more subtle means to keep them in their place. Parents no longer say "no" to Elliott or Courtney because, well, generally speaking, you just don't say "no" any more. It's like your boss: he doesn't say "no" – he says "maybe." Your loan officer is "going to study your file" before spitting out (with regret, but you insisted on getting an answer), "I am afraid that it won't be possible." Nobody in the world says "no" any more. We have been everywhere, seen everything, explored the remotest planets and the most secret parts of the body. We have even shone light on the reproduction process. On desire? On the unconscious? Well, not really, yet, but the neuroscientists seem to be working on it. Is there anyone who still says "no" to us? The terrorist, maybe. In fact he doesn't just settle for "no": he puts "fuck" before it for good measure.

So if you want to be a "good parent" – at least the way society sees it – you have to be neutral. He wants to decorate his room with a giant Megadeth poster? She collects Diddl stickers and puts them up all over the place? Or she always eats the same foods, refuses raw vegetables, and his favourite dinner is a McDonald's Happy Meal? Your face must remain perfectly calm, show no value judgment, because that could "traumatize" the poor kid. Everything is permissible; kids must be able to "carve their own identity." In today's world, it won't do to yell, "Get these eyesores out of your room! As long as I'm paying the rent, I'll make the decisions around here." Or, "What kind of crap is this! Anybody who's interested in stuff as stupid as this can't be the flesh of my flesh; some gene must have mutated." Parents, like managers, must stay calm under all circumstances, and demonstrate their capacity for listening.

Above all, there can be no violence. To strike a child has become unthinkable. In Scandinavia, corporal punishment within the family is forbidden by law. A book like *Le bébé de Monsieur Laurent*, by the prolific and provocative Roland Topor – an absurd and hilarious story about a baby nailed to a door – would probably never see the light of day now (and it has not been reissued). As for me, not being very skilful with a hammer, I have, I admit it, slapped my son. I know these words are likely to be shocking to the sensitive reader and to earn me a denunciation down at the Child Protection Agency. But here are the facts. My son was tearing all over the municipal library, shouting and disturbing everyone, and refusing to listen to my reprimands. I slapped him. Evil had possessed me. A well-intentioned woman explained to me that it was monstrous to hit children. When I told her to mind her own ass, she threatened to call the police. Having kids means running a lot of risks, both with the authorities and with public opinion.

32.
Parenthood is a sad, sweet song

Always happy, cheerful, smiling. Even when you are getting ragged on by your colleagues, or your favourite uncle has just died. At work, people who deal with the public are supposed to demonstrate continuous enthusiasm (on this score, we have a long way to go, and I don't know whether to laugh or cry about it).

It's the same at home. They keep telling parents that you have to "keep the child active" right from the earliest years. You're expected to discuss things with them, to cry "Bravo!" when they babble, to get them to play, to read books to them from birth, to sing them songs while doing "this is the way" with your hands, to transform mealtime into a "convivial and agreeable moment," to show joy and interest at the sound of a burp or the contents of a diaper. To pull off a performance like this, you have to be either an idiot or full of Prozac. Will seeing their parents play the fool all day long make kids more intelligent? I have my doubts. It might render them completely stupid. Could this explain the famous and hackneyed "academic decline" of students that has obsessed so many pedagogues since . . . antiquity?

When the kids get a little older, you're supposed to be an example to them. That can be hard on a daily basis. Stuffing yourself with Nutella sandwiches on the couch, smoking pot when you get home from work, guzzling a good (or not so good) wine in bed – these are not proper examples for children. Dragging yourself around the house with greasy hair and a dirty nightgown is also not the kind of example likely to turn them into responsible and positive adults. In such an environment, how are they going to "pull themselves together"?

Bursting into tears in front of them because Julianna has just played some trick, or because you didn't get your promotion – that is not recommended. To say nothing of having a fight with your partner, along with the attendant reproaches and screaming – the kind of scenes that condemn your child to years on the analyst's couch, if not to alcoholism and juvenile delinquency.

The hardest thing of all is maintaining an antiseptic tone when talking about the world into which they have just arrived. But you have to try, all the same. You have to talk about "values" (honesty, being considerate of others, keeping your word), even if these are precisely the things you must not respect if you want to climb the ladder in a world of rivalry and competition. You are urged to tell them about gender equality while buying them anti-sexist toys (dolls for the boys, chemistry sets for the girls, books that have been cleansed of the stereotypes of bygone days), even if there is no real equality in your own home. Never forget that parents are the *missi dominici** of the Empire of the Good. The major-domos of Yes-Yes Land. Conformity and moral clarity are essential. Detachment and skepticism are frowned upon. Are you naturally pessimistic, even at times a bit depressed? Do you sometimes question the meaning of

---

* "Envoys of the Lord," emissaries sent by medieval Frankish kings to supervise provincial administration. (Ed.)

life, the sense of the word *democratic*? Work on yourself to get rid of this deadly negativity. When you have children, you must put them on the right track and force yourself under every circumstance to be positive, talk friendly, talk *citizen*.

No harshness. Neutrality. Compassion – worthy of the evening news. Soft music studded with positive language, like a political speech. That is what society expects of parents, even if a lot of them fail because the burden is so heavy. If despite this book you still want to become a parent, you have to start practising now, in front of the mirror, because it's real work. I'd advise signing up for an acting course, perhaps one called "Always put on a happy face in front of your children and give them a positive image of the society in which they live." Being a parent is no child's game: it's an actor's game.

33.
Motherhood is a trap for women

The cult of the child weighs heavily upon women. The modern woman must be a mother, an employee, and a friend all at once. Preferably thin. And you have to admit, that's a lot to ask. On top of that, women do 80 per cent of the housework. When school lets out, you mostly see women there; the same at parents' night, or at the pediatrician's when a kid has bronchitis or chickenpox. For many women, motherhood means getting home early at night to look after the kids, missing those important meetings that are held after 7 p.m. (they are always held after 7 p.m.), turning down or not even applying for jobs that are more interesting but too time consuming.

If until recently women have held such a minor position in the history of human culture, it is quite simply because they've been handed the dirty work, having to go through the pain of childbirth and to raise the brood. Before the 20th century, there were very few examples of women writers, musicians, painters, or scientists. Maybe making children was a substitute: "creating" a human being was, perhaps, seen as the equivalent of creating a work of art. As a substitute? Or as a last resort. "Creation" by way of maternity is available to all: it is a real democracy of the uterus. Some women have preferred to express themselves through a more demanding route. Hannah Arendt, Simone Weil, Virginia Woolf, and Simone de Beauvoir did not have children. For de Beauvoir it was a choice: she believed that you could not be both a good mother and an intellectual. In *The Second Sex*, she characterized motherhood as an obstacle to transcendence.

Can you have an original thought while wiping bums, giving bottles, and listening to multiplication tables? The jury is still out. There's no question that the prosaic and exhausting tasks that come with mother-hood are a dead weight on the deployment of the giant wings of thought. Are women the victims of an unjust order of things set out by men? Or are they the victims of their own children, who provide so many excuses for not creating or accomplishing anything? That's all there is to it: who knows what I might have become if I hadn't had kids, if I had been less wrapped up in running the house, doing the shopping, serving the meals? I confess that I'm just waiting for one thing: getting my kids through school so that I can finally have some time for my own little creative activities. I'll be fifty then. Later on, when I'm grown up, life will really begin.

34.
Motherhood or success: Pick one

Working mothers are a majority now in Europe. That may be progress, but it is not necessarily a promotion because very few of those women are professionally suc-cessful, despite social policies that favour families with children. French women are certainly the envy of the whole world (daycares, state subsidies, generous mater-nity leave . . .), but the wage gap between men and women still averages about 27 per cent. The time that the poor *merdeuf* spends with her kids, making meals, vacuuming, and telling silly stories, is time she does not spend at work. According to one economist, women who have to take care of children earn some €100,000 to €150,000 euros ($150,000 to $225,000) less than they could have, averaged out over their whole careers.

And while 80 per cent are working, only 30 per cent ever make it into important positions – a little better than in Germany and especially Italy, but not as good as in the U.K. Do you know many female CEOs, press barons, members of parliament? The famous glass ceiling stops women from getting the top jobs, and those jobs do have one great advantage: the higher you rise, the fewer idiots there are above you. It is not astonishing that biographies of successful women never fail to note the number of children they've had: those are obstacles they've had to overcome in order to make something interesting out of their lives. It's a bit like running a marathon with a five-kilogram weight (per child) on each foot.

Furthermore, motherhood is often the equivalent of a part time job that offers no prospects and no hope of promotion: 31 per cent of today's women work part time. Of those who are working, many have few qualifications and are in the lower-echelon service industries, the public sector, or, at best, the education system. A lot of underpaid jobs do allow time for one's parental duties. For women the implicit deal is this: "The job is not great, but you have time to look after your children, so what are you complaining about?"

As for the less qualified, generous financial assistance has clearly persuaded them to quit the labour market.

And don't talk to me about these "new fathers" who get a lot more involved in the home than previous male generations did. True, they know how to change a diaper and bottle-feed the baby. But that doesn't mean that they sacrifice their careers. The proof: when men become fathers, their professional activities increase and they devote more time to their jobs – the opposite of women. Studies show that men who have brilliant careers are often the fathers of families loaded with children, while the most successful women are often childless. There is no doubt about it: children are an accelerator for the one, a millstone for the other. In the Zapatero government of Spain at the start of 2007, there were eight men and eight women; the former had twenty-four children among them, the latter only five. (Relax, reader: this is not a math problem for schoolchildren.) You want gender equality? Start by not having children.

35.
When the child appears, the father disappears

Fathers are not what they used to be. He's no longer the head of the household, by divine right, whom all obey without a murmur. We don't know what happened to that stereotype; he slipped out on the sly, hand in hand with the Stakhanovite,* of whom we also hear no more. Today's father is usually a slightly bald chap of forty, well endowed with love handles, somewhat dis-illusioned with the world and with himself. He can hardly say a word about his day when he comes home at night because the kids cut him off all the time, and he was totally bored at work anyway.

A lot of sociologists and shrinks yammer on about the death of the father and the decline of authority. In fact, it is not the father who is dead; it is his power to make others jump that has disappeared. Not that we're living in a permissive society – quite the opposite; but today, obedience is imposed on us by the system, not by individuals. In the '70s, the American philosopher Christopher Lasch, somewhat ahead of his time, put forward the idea that his era was characterized by a "paternalism without any fathers." Don't hold that against the fathers of today though; they still want to be cool and open-minded, but without assuming any sort of authority where their word is law. Meanwhile, paternalism is thriving in the form of the welfare state, a protective social system, and a bureaucracy that deems itself benevolent. For example: in the big bureaucracies, nobody ever reproaches you directly; they just wait for

---

* A Soviet Russian term of approval for an outstandingly productive worker. (Ed.)

you to impose upon yourself what the organization intended in the first place. And so power is becoming completely impersonal and no longer requires an authority figure to make people behave. The steamroller runs by itself. Wicked, isn't it?

There are no fathers left, only progenitors. And there's more. Becoming a father means a man's role is reduced to (just barely) supporting his family. A man no longer *decides* to become a father. Fifty years ago, it was the men who turned women into mothers, often against their wishes. Nowadays the power relationship is reversed: only motherhood is voluntary, not fatherhood. A man becomes a father only when he is accepted as such. Women today have the upper hand with the children: whether or not they'll be born, who is going to raise them, whose name they will have. Women no longer hold men by the balls but by the belly – their own.

And while the divorced father, in the name of equal recognition, may fight a justice system that deprives him of his children, the married woman is struggling to have more balanced domestic and parental responsibilities within the family. Is that unfair? Yes, perhaps. But genuine equality between the sexes is probably an illusion. After all, since it is the women who perform all the key duties in the household, it's pretty reasonable that they should be the decision-makers too, isn't it? The one who does the work makes the decisions. If that logic were applied to the business world and to politics, this would be one hell of a different world.

36.
Today's child is the perfect child: Welcome to the best of all possible worlds

Being a parent means closely guarding the health of our dear kids. Probably because of the constant watch that is kept over them, children enjoy flourishing good health – no more tuberculosis, no more cholera. Infant mortality has never been so low . . . nor have we ever been so fearful for their lives. A lot of parents rush to the pediatrician or overwhelm emergency rooms at the least little sign of a cold. The great plagues may have been eradicated, but others have taken their place. New diseases have multiplied over the last twenty years, from sleep disorders to emotional development problems, by way of allergies, speech retardation, obesity, school phobia. . . .

The scourge of parents is the hyperactive child, a newly invented malady. A few years ago, a kid like that was just a pain in the ass. He awakes at sunrise with a bugle call, and throughout the day, one idiocy follows another; he talks non-stop and yells at the least little annoyance. But what is even more worrisome is that it's hard to distinguish the hyperactive child from any other kid. He's just a contemporary child, but worse. Just *worse*. It is the "just" part that makes the situation intolerable. Some kids simply accumulate defects. And in that great lottery of the chromosomes, you might just find yourself saddled with a hyperactive *obese* child!

To keep disease at bay, you have to protect kids from themselves. Explain everything – never mind what – and always in a calm and responsible tone of voice. Diligently persuade them to eat green beans and tomatoes and not just pizza and hamburgers smothered in ketchup. I've seen parents tearing their hair out because their kid "doesn't eat." (But he's still alive, how can that be?) Since you can't use force any more (that just isn't done), you have to deploy all your diplomatic resources and patience to get them to take a mouthful here, a mouthful there, of fruit and vegetables.

Usually parents know how to do this, a stick in one hand and a carrot in the other, since lots of people deal with the parents themselves in this way – politicians, managers, even some doctors. Isn't an adult just an irresponsible kid who's been surrounded by hygienic, charitable, humanist, and protective programs? Adults have to be watched over too: tell them not to smoke, explain the dangers of alcohol. . . . All for their well-being and for the well-being of the community. To educate people for citizenship, you have to use instruction and pedagogy, a word you keep hearing everywhere.

Only pedagogy can stop demagogy. Do you take us for children? When I hear the word *pedagogy*, I get out my revolver (I mean my pen). Pedagogy is the art of controlling people without their catching on.

Children must be healthy, well integrated, well adjusted to school. The pressure weighing on them is enormous. Of course, we'll need some payback for all this stuff we give them – the toys, the time we've spent with them, the hopes we've invested in them. They will pay for all that, and pay a lot. To justify all this excess of care and anguish of which they are the object, the children will have to perform, both physically and mentally. And to that end we have to consult a speech therapist if they resist learning to talk, an orthodontist to straighten their teeth, a nutritionist to help them lose weight, a psychologist if they don't appear to be "fulfilled." Only children from whom little is expected (like me, and my parents were no monsters for all that) will ever know and appreciate, when they grow up, how free that makes them: whatever they do, they will never be a disappointment.

Do you want to be sure you have a healthy child who is prepared to string out, like pearls, those forty-two years of pension contributions that will bring in the one genuine freedom of the salaried worker – retirement? Thanks to progress in genetics, you can get a pre-implantation genetic diagnosis (otherwise known as PGD, since without the acronym, which looks good, the term itself looks silly and vague). This is a genetic analysis that shows, during or even before pregnancy, whether an embryo might be vulnerable to certain hereditary illnesses or deformations. The purpose? To have healthy children. Ones that last, like Duracell batteries. Guaranteed on the invoice. Defective child? Scrap it. Abnormal? Somewhere else, not in our house. Mozart, who probably had Tourette's syndrome, would be considered a deviant today, not worth keeping alive. So far, in France, only thirty-four fetuses have been brought to term after PGD, but you can be sure that that number will soon skyrocket. And one day every single child will be flawless – no disease, no cancer, no schizophrenia, no depression. So, will their lives be flawless too? And will the world they live in be flawless? I somehow doubt it.

37.
Danger, child ahead

Children are dangerous. They can bring on lawsuits and cost you your freedom (admittedly already pretty relative). Because these innocent little creatures are quite ready to denounce their parents and turn them over to the authorities without a second thought. Keep in mind that in a totalitarian regime, it is the kids who get enlisted first. The classic example is the good little communists who denounce their parents to the secret police for ideological incorrectness. Minor examples can be found closer to home. In 2001, in a dismal northern town called Outreau, where there's not much to do, eighteen people were imprisoned after being denounced as pedophiles by a number of children and spent one to three years in jail. One committed suicide. It was a judicial error, of course: the little darlings had lied, advised by some underqualified "experts" and believed by incompetent judges.

At first we are outraged by Outreau, and then frightened. That could happen to any of us parents! A shiver runs up the spine. In fact, it happened to a friend of mine: his thirteen-year-old daughter, in a mood one day, told them at school that her father had tied her to the bed. The police got involved, the parents were called in for interrogation, and it took them months to establish their innocence. (It has to be noted here that Ségolène Royal's 1997 directive instructed school authorities that they should never doubt the word of children who claim to have been abused.)

Why should a child's word be believed over that of an adult? Because it is the truth – the potential victim is necessarily innocent. This is not far from the myth of original innocence. And of course children are the eighth wonder of the world in the eyes of their parents, who are convinced that a lot of evil-minded adults are prowling around them with hateful sexual outrages in mind. Would Nabokov's erotic novel *Lolita* ever get published these days? Not sure. Our world is haunted by the child molester as the symbol of absolute evil, worse than the SS. The incarnation of the most abject rapist-killer is Marc Dutroux, a monster guilty of numerous murders and rapes. It is Dutroux who's really behind the Outreau outrage. This is a kind of wide-spectrum precautionary principle: since a Dutroux lurks within each of us, let's keep all adults under control.

You don't even have to be accused by your child. Just taking her photograph can get you into trouble with the law. Iconophiles watch out! In 2005, a Dutch artist, Kiki Lamers, got an eight-month suspended prison sentence and a fine of €5,000 for having taken nude photographs of her own children to use for her paintings. The protection of children justifies repression? We must be dreaming! But the nightmare continued when, in 2006, the director of the École des Beaux Arts in Paris, Henry-Claude Cousseau, was investigated for having organized a show in 2000 called Presumed Innocent: Contemporary Art and Childhood. What violence or pornography or indignities were there in this show featuring the cream of contemporary artists – Christian Boltanski, Jeff Koons, Cindy Sherman, and others? Annette Messager unleashed the fury of the self-styled defenders of childhood with a work called *Children with Their Eyes Scratched Out*: newspaper pictures of children, their eyes scratched out with a ballpoint pen. It leaves you speechless. Are you serious,

Inspector? I bet that one of these days clinical echograms are going to take the place of porn and be traded under the table. Basically, it's the same principle: everything should be visible, right down to the bones. No way will we let any mystery skulk in the corner.

38.
Why wear yourself out
for a future that
doesn't include you?

You are going to have your child on your hands for decades – a burden from which you will find it difficult to escape. My advice? If you really want to be host to a parasite, get a gigolo. It's more fun and at least you'll know what you're getting into. You'll try to tell me that in twenty years the world will have become more hospitable to young children; not likely, given that things have gotten steadily worse for them for a whole generation.

Here's something to think about. Children are the embodiment of psychoanalyst Jacques Lacan's "object a": that is, at one and the same time a marvel and a piece of garbage. And in the past, they were indeed a little of each. For a long time, children were seen as parasites – not always desired; far from it, their existence itself rather uncertain. One is reminded somewhat of the value that Montaigne, in his *Essays*, attributed to his own children, almost all of whom died young. "I prefer a good book to a child," he said, in effect. It is true that every newborn is the result of its parents' desire, but also that the child will be a parasite to its family and relatives for years. Today, children are invariably seen as miracles. This is not necessarily good news, because the youths they cannot help becoming are destined to end up as failures and outsiders. Youth aren't supposed to introduce anything new into the world; the young person is supposed to conform to the established ideal of youth. And we see too that many celebrities refuse to grow up, Michael Jackson in the lead, or those two little rebels, Brad Pitt and Johnny Depp.

So the coddled child is destined to become a youthful outsider. The world loves that beauty, that youth, that freshness – but, gorgeous object, be handsome and shut up. Youths who live in countries that are too rich, too cultured, where everything has already been done or at least attempted, feel that they are not appreciated for who they are. Since we no longer have wars or colonies – the traditional dumping grounds for idle youth – the kid has nothing to do but twiddle his thumbs and wait for a better day. Of course, he has the right to make love, which was not the case until the 1960s: don't forget that the events of May 1968 started because the boys wanted access to the girls' dormitories. Enjoy life, of course, but forget about having any opinion about anything, never mind trying to change things.

France, like other baby-loving countries, is actually not very hospitable to youth, who can expect mass unemployment, precarious jobs, and insufficient housing until at least the age of thirty. In the twenty to twenty-five age group, the youth unemployment rate is shockingly high, and those few who have managed to "insert themselves" have all the flexibility that France doesn't want at any price: 87 per cent of these young people have the most insecure kind of employment – read, "shit jobs." Poorer than their parents were at that age, even if they have more diplomas, these loser babies are a burden to the unemployment centres, potential delinquents, or, at the very least, socially disadvantaged.

The system needs people with no history, no clear or secure identity, who live fragmented in a permanent present. Your urchins, soon to be among the un-employed, will go from day to day, living a life with no purpose, no goal or dream except to be "assimilated." Security, certainty, self-determination – they won't even remember what these words mean. They'll have no reason to live. Faster, always faster, into the trash can. They'll reflect a way of life where nothing lasts, where things that are useful today will be the next day's rubbish. Unsure of tomorrow, facing the anguish of the future, they'll be forced to get through life without ever understanding the vague rules of this society that purposely confuses them. There are no longer any instruction books for people who want to plan their route: if you have children, you will have nothing to pass on to them, no recipe, no "how-to" that is worth anything. It's not surprising that the number of young adults suffering from depression has doubled in the last twelve years.* De Gaulle used to say that old age was a kind of shipwreck; today, that describes youth.

39.
There are too many children in the world

Too much stuff, too many cafés, too many shops, too many brands of organic whole wheat bread, too many people. The world's population is now 6.5 billion; in 2030, it will be close to 8 billion. The poorest have the most children – the birthrate in so-called developed countries has dropped below the magic number of 2.1 per woman, considered to be the replacement rate (zero population growth).

Nonetheless, the planet is not overcrowded; if the entire populations of China and India were moved to the North American continent, it wouldn't be any more

---

* According to the Joseph Rowntree Foundation, quoted by John Carvel in "Depression on the rise among the young," *The Guardian*, November 27, 2002.

crowded than Holland, Belgium, or England. The problem is excess pollution. The relatively small population of the developed countries consumes two-thirds of the world's energy resources. In fact, it's not that there are too many people on the planet – there are just too many *rich* people.

We are the planet's freeloaders, and we keep increasing our consumption. Does it really make any sense for us to have children who will consume even more, and always to the detriment of the world's poorest? Nobody needs our kids, because we and they are the spoiled brats of a planet that is heading straight for annihilation. If you live in Europe or America, then having kids is immoral. Always wasting more limited resources for a voracious lifestyle, always overspending, always guzzling gas, always more destructive of the environment.

To have a kid in a rich country is not the act of a citizen. The State should be helping those who decide *not* to have children: less unemployment, less congestion, fewer wars. Try for a second to imagine your country with several million fewer people – less greenhouse gas, fewer lineups to rent condos, fewer traffic jams on the highways on the weekend or lines at the cinema to see *Borat* or long wait times for surgery. A genuine land of milk and honey.

Some European countries have been smart enough to curtail their birthrates. Forecasts for 2050 see

Germany with only 73 million (80 million today), Italy with 50 instead of 58 million, Spain with 35 instead of 40 million. Want to go and visit the great mosque of Cordova without getting stuck in a mob of tourists? Or see the Sistine Chapel in peace and quiet? Tomorrow that might be possible. Let's copy those countries. Let's put more effort into "de-natality." *No Kids* is a destination we could reasonably get to if we stick together, on guard together: if no sperm finds its way to an ovum.

40.
Reject the absurd ten commandments of the "good" parent.

1. Your children are more important than you, than your work, than you as a couple, than any other child, than all the adults living or dead in the world you live in.
2. You must teach them the gentle values (tolerance of others, honesty) that nobody respects and that are useless for getting ahead socially or making money – they are, in fact, obstacles.
3. You must desire their "well-being." Nobody knows what that really means, but maybe they will, some day, if you work really hard for them. If children seem unhappy these days, it's

because their parents don't do enough for them,
that's all.

4. Keep them busy at all times, in as many ways
as possible. It's a huge undertaking, but you
must undertake it, so that they will be stimu-
lated and *fulfilled*.

5. You must be an example to them. No drugs,
no drinking, no orgies at home. No bad taste.
No inappropriate humour. Ideally, no tears or
arguments or sorrow, though sometimes those
are unavoidable.

6. You will protect your children from the many
dangers that threaten them, since they are
potential victims. Whatever they do, they are
neither responsible nor guilty. (They always
tell the truth.)

7. You must help your children "adapt" and move
around and be "flexible" in this world of
change. Don't forget – someday they will be,
above all, tourists.

8. You must never hit them. You will neither
punish nor scold. School and society will
look after that, cramming them into little
pigeonholes.

9. You will talk to them as much as possible, and
explain everything, no matter what.

10. You will always be positive. You will tell them
about the world they will live in when they are

grown, a world of citizens, pluralistic, global-
ized, against discrimination; then they'll be
eager to grow up. But not too fast, because
childhood is still the only true paradise.

Conclusion

CHILDREN? NO THANKS

No kids, thanks. It's better that way. "De-natality" is our only hope. Women, the future of our planet depends on you. The last freedom is to *choose not to*. Like Bartleby, Herman Melville's subversive hero who spread disorder in the workplace through his recalcitrance, and who quite clearly had no children.

"I would prefer not to" is the most deconstructionist expression of negative thinking. It is the refuge of all those who are not so naive as to think they might have solutions to propose or the cynicism to make others think that they have. It is the call to arms of those who wonder why you have to say yes, with enthusiasm and goodwill, to this constant litany of the Best of All Possible Worlds that they're selling us as if it were the triumph of centuries of progress and humanism.

I would prefer . . . not to have children. Not to work. Not to watch the news on television. Not to be part of this economic competition.

You too – you could decide that you would "prefer not to." *Not-to's* of the world, my sisters and brothers, let us stay disunited, skeptical, and, if possible, without descendants.

WITHDRAWN

Corinne Maier is the bestselling author of *Hello Laziness*. She lives in Brussels with her husband and two children, where she is a practicing psychoanalyst.

WITHDRAWN